GOLDEN HOUR
**The Handbook of
Advanced Pediatric
Life Support**

GOLDEN HOUR
THE HANDBOOK OF ADVANCED PEDIATRIC LIFE SUPPORT

From the
Division of Pediatric Intensive Care
and the Pediatric Trauma Service
of The Johns Hopkins Hospital

Editors

David G. Nichols, M.D.
Myron Yaster, M.D.
Dorothy G. Lappe, R.N., M.S.
James R. Buck, M.D.

Medical Illustrations by:
Timothy H. Phelps, M.S., A.M.I.

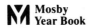
St. Louis   Baltimore   Boston   Chicago   London   Philadelphia   Sydney   Toronto

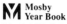

M Mosby
Year Book
Dedicated to Publishing Excellence

Sponsoring Editor: James Shanahan
Associate Managing Editor, Manuscript Services: Deborah Thorp
Production Coordinator: Nancy C. Baker
Proofroom Manager: Barbara Kelly

NOTICE

Every effort has been made to ensure that the drug dosage schedules herein are accurate and in accord with the standards accepted at the time of publication. However, as new research and experience broaden our knowledge, changes in treatment and drug therapy occur. Therefore, the reader is advised to check the product information sheet included in the package of each drug he plans to administer to be certain that changes have not been made in the recommended dose or in the contraindications. This is of particular importance in regard to new or infrequently used drugs.

1 2 3 4 5 6 7 8 9 0   CL/MA   95 94 93 92 91

Library of Congress Cataloging-in-Publication Data
Golden hour: the handbook of advanced pediatric life support / David
    G. Nichols . . . [et al.].
       p. cm.
    Includes bibliographical references.
    Includes index.
    ISBN 0-8151-6395-9
    1. Pediatric emergencies. 2. Life support systems (Critical care)
I. Nichols, David G. (David Gregory), 1951-
    [DNLM: 1. Emergencies—in infancy & childhood. 2. Life Support
Care—in infancy & childhood. 3. Wounds and Injuries—in infancy &
childhood. WS 200 G595]
    RJ370.G65 1991
    618.92′0025—dc20
    DNLM/DLC   91-6363
    for Library of Congress   CIP

PREFACE

"He who saves a life saves the world."

The Talmud

Few experiences in life match the exhilaration and terror that accompany the emergency management of a critically ill or injured child. The initial resuscitation usually occurs in a tumultuous, chaotic, and highly charged atmosphere in which there is little time to think or deliberate on management options. Success is dependent on a team approach utilizing well rehearsed, systematic management protocols that can be implemented within the first, or **"golden,"** hour of presentation.

In 1982, Dr. J. Alex Haller and Dr. Frank R. Gioia developed and instituted the original Advanced Pediatric Life Support Course at the Johns Hopkins Hospital that continues to this day. The faculty they assembled to teach these management protocols and skills are the authors and editors of this book.

The editors wish to express their thanks to the emergency medical technicians, paramedics, nurses, pediatricians, emergency medicine physicians, surgeons, and intensivists who have developed, refined, and instituted the protocols described in this book. Additionally, this book would not have been possible without the tireless efforts of Dr. Michael Bezman and the assistance of Drs. Aaron L. Zuckerberg and Mark A. Helfaer. Finally, the editors wish to express their thanks to Dr. Mark C. Rogers and Dr. Frank A. Oski whose dedication to the welfare of children and commitment to excellence have provided the impetus that has made this book possible.

David G. Nichols, M.D.
Myron Yaster, M.D.
Dorothy G. Lappe, R.N., M.S.
James R. Buck, M.D.

CONTRIBUTORS

Alice D. Ackerman, M.D.
Assistant Professor of Pediatrics
University of Maryland Medical System
Baltimore, Maryland

Bonnie L. Beaver, M.D.
Assistant Professor of Pediatric Surgery
University of Maryland Medical System
Baltimore, Maryland

Ivor D. Berkowitz, M.B.B.Ch.
Assistant Professor of Anesthesiology/Critical Care
Medicine and Pediatrics
Johns Hopkins University
Baltimore, Maryland

Michael Bezman, M.D.
Research Assistant
Department of Anesthesiology/Critical Care Medicine
Johns Hopkins University
Baltimore, Maryland

James R. Buck, M.D.
Assistant Professor of Pediatric Surgery
Assistant Chief of Service, Sinai Hospital
Baltimore, Maryland

Benjamin S. Carson, M.D.
Assistant Professor of Neurosurgery, Oncology, and Pediatrics
Johns Hopkins University
Baltimore, Maryland

Jayant K. Deshpande, M.D.
Assistant Professor of Anesthesiology/Critical Care
Medicine and Pediatrics
Johns Hopkins University
Baltimore, Maryland

J. Alex Haller, Jr., M.D.
Robert Garrett Professor of Pediatric Surgery
Professor of Pediatrics and Emergency Medicine
Johns Hopkins University
Baltimore, Maryland

Steven E. Haun, M.D.
Assistant Professor of Pediatrics
University of Ohio
Columbus, Ohio

Mark A. Helfaer, M.D.
Assistant Professor of Anesthesiology/Critical Care Medicine
Johns Hopkins University
Baltimore, Maryland

Dorothy G. Lappe, R.N., M.S.
Nurse Manager, Pediatric Intensive Care Unit
Johns Hopkins Hospital
Baltimore, Maryland

David G. Nichols, M.D.
Assistant Professor of Anesthesiology/Critical Care
Medicine and Pediatrics
Johns Hopkins University
Baltimore, Maryland

Mark C. Rogers, M.D.
Professor and Chairman
Department of Anesthesiology/Critical Care Medicine
Professor of Pediatrics
Johns Hopkins University
Baltimore, Maryland

L.R. Scherer, III, M.D.
Assistant Professor of Pediatric Surgery, Pediatrics,
Anesthesiology/Critical Care Medicine
Johns Hopkins University
Baltimore, Maryland

Charles L. Schleien, M.D.
Assistant Professor of Pediatrics
University of Miami Medical Center
Miami, Florida

Paul D. Sponseller, M.D.
Assistant Professor of Orthopaedic Surgery
Johns Hopkins University
Baltimore, Maryland

Randall C. Wetzel, M.B., B.S., F.C.C.M.
Associate Professor of Anesthesiology/Critical Care
Medicine and Pediatrics
Johns Hopkins University
Baltimore, Maryland

Lawrence S. Wissow, M.D.
Assistant Professor of Pediatrics
Johns Hopkins University
Baltimore, Maryland

Myron Yaster, M.D.
Associate Professor of Anesthesiology/Critical Care
Medicine and Pediatrics
Johns Hopkins University

CONTENTS

LISTING OF TABLES

LISTING OF FIGURES

Chapter 1
INITIAL ASSESSMENT

I.   INTRODUCTION

The management of a critically ill or injured child requires a systematic, well rehearsed approach that can be instituted almost reflexively (Figure 1-1). One must be able to identify the management priorities for stabilization of the patient even before a complete history and physical examination have been obtained. Indeed, definitive therapy may not be possible until resuscitation and stabilization are complete. Finally, success is only possible if the unique anatomic, physiologic and pathophysiologic responses of children are understood by the resuscitation team.

II.   PRIMARY SURVEY

A.   Definition

The primary survey involves the first evaluation of the patient's condition at which time the life threatening problems are identified. A hierarchy of management priorities for resuscitation and stabilization is established.

B.   Steps in a Primary Survey

The primary survey is designed to assess the following items in the order listed.

1.   Airway
2.   **Breathing** (ventilation)
3.   **Circulation** (hemorrhage control)
4.   **Disability** (neurologic examination)
5.   **Exposure** (temperature)

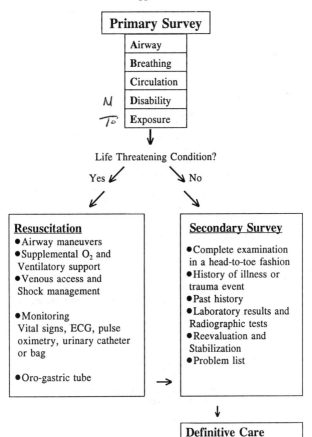

Figure 1-1. Algorithm of the initial assessment of pediatric patient

C. **Airway**

The goals of airway management are:
1. Recognition and relief of obstruction.
2. Prevention of aspiration of gastric contents.
3. Promotion of adequate gas exchange.
4. Further detailed information regarding pediatric airway management is discussed in *Chapter 2*.

D. **Breathing**

1. Once the patient's airway is established, the child must be observed for adequate breathing. Air exchange may be deficient from central causes such as apnea or from abnormal chest wall dynamics such as a tension pneumothorax. The cause of the problem should be treated immediately.

2. Methods to augment ventilation
    a. Mouth-to-mouth, mouth-to-nose breathing
    b. Mask-bag ventilation
    c. Endotracheal intubation
    d. Cricothyrotomy (needle or surgical).

3. Emergency breathing techniques are further described in *Chapter 6* and *Chapter 2*.

E. **Circulation**

1. The adequacy of circulation is assessed by noting the quality, rate, and regularity of the pulse centrally and peripherally. Capillary refill and blood pressure are determined. Note: blood pressure is one of the least sensitive measures of adequate circulation in children. Compromised circulation may exist despite a normal blood pressure in children. Normal hemodynamic values for children are given in Table 1-1.

2. Circulatory support during the primary survey may require:

   a. Control of active hemorrhage
   b. Intravenous fluid, crystalloid/blood
   c. MAST suit application
   d. External cardiac massage
   e. Defibrillation

3. More comprehensive information regarding shock is discussed in *Chapter 5*.

TABLE 1-1. Ranges of Vital Sign Parameters

Age	Mean Pulse Rate/min	Respiratory Rate/min	Systolic/Diastolic Blood Pressure (mm Hg)
Premature	125±50	30-60	35-56 systolic
Newborn	140±50	30-60	75/50
1-6 months	130±45	30-40	80/46
6-12 months	115±40	24-30	96/65
12-24 months	110±40	20-30	99/65
2-6 years	105±35	20-25	100/60
6-12 years	95±30	16-20	110/60
Over 12 yrs of age	82±25	12-16	120/60

F. Disability

    1.   A rapid screening neurologic evaluation is performed as part of the primary survey. This includes assessment of pupillary response, level of consciousness, and notation of any localized findings.

    2.   Detailed explanation of neurologic assessment is included in *Chapter 9* and in *Chapter 15*.

G. Exposure

    1.   Passive heat loss

        A complete physical examination requires undressing the patient. Because of their large surface to body mass ratio, children cool rapidly, particularly when homeostatic mechanisms may be disrupted by disease states.

    2.   Hypo- and hyperthermia are discussed in *Chapter 13*.

III. SECONDARY SURVEY

A. Definition

The secondary survey includes a detailed physical examination. Also included are a history of the illness or trauma event, a brief past history, indicated laboratory and radiographic studies which lead to a specific diagnosis or list of problems requiring further attention.

B. Head

    1.   The face is examined for

        a.   Evidence of maxillofacial trauma by

            (1) palpation of bony prominences;

            (2) presence of bloody or cerebral spinal fluid discharge from nose, mouth, or ears;

        b.   Dehydration

            (1) sunken eyes and/or fontanelle,

        (2)   dry mouth mucosa;

    c.   Poisoning and metabolic problems
        (1)   odor from mouth,
        (2)   discoloration of mucosa.

2.   The eyes are examined for pupillary size and reaction, fundal appearance and vision if possible.

3.   The scalp is carefully examined for laceration or hematoma. Specific signs of basilar skull fractures include Battle sign (ecchymoses behind the ear) and "raccoon eyes" (ecchymoses around both eyes).

C. Neck

The neck is palpated for obvious signs of fractures and midline position of the trachea.

D. Chest

1.   The chest is inspected for adequacy of respiratory excursion, asymmetry of respiration or for the presence of a flail segment.

2.   The chest is then carefully palpated and the lung fields and heart are auscultated.

3.   Thoracic trauma is discussed in *Chapter 16*; asthma and respiratory failure in *Chapter 4*.

E. Abdomen

1.   The initial examination of the abdomen includes inspection for ease of abdominal wall movement with respiration, gentle palpation for localized guarding or mass, and auscultation for bowel sounds.

2.   The flanks are observed for hematoma and palpated.

3.   Serial examinations are often needed to establish a correct diagnosis.

4.   In females of childbearing age, pregnancy and pregnancy related problems must be investigated.

F. Pelvis
  1. The bony prominences of the pelvis are palpated for tenderness or instability.
  2. The perineum is examined for laceration, hematoma, active bleeding or discharge (inflammatory). Child abuse is discussed in *Chapter 14.*

G. Rectum
  A rectal examination is indicated if pelvic fracture, bowel pathology, or child abuse is suspected.

H. Extremities
  1. The extremities are examined for signs of abrasion, contusion or hematoma formation. Soft tissue injuries are discussed in *Chapter 19.*
  2. Bony instability is noted and a neurovascular examination is performed on all extremities.
  3. Orthopaedic injuries are discussed in *Chapter 18.*

I. Neurologic examination
  1. Include motor, sensory, cranial nerve and level of consciousness in an in-depth examination.
  2. The tympanic membranes and the nose are examined for signs of basilar skull fracture.
  3. The fundi are examined if this has not occurred yet.
  4. A numerical evaluation may aid in subsequent examination and the modified Glasgow coma score is recommended here (see *Chapter 9*).
  5. The presence of spinal cord trauma is noted (flaccidity, hypotension without tachycardia, absent reflexes).
  6. Neurologic assessment is further discussed in *Chapter 9 and 15.*

J. Bony Structures of the Back

The patient with obvious spinal cord trauma is immobilized on a back board and with a cervical collar. If there is no obvious spinal cord injury and paralysis, the patient should be turned gently to examine the back for evidence of trauma.

K. Skin

Skin should be examined simultaneously during all previous steps.

1. Bruises

    The color and size may be suggestive of trauma or coagulopathy.

2. Rash

    Hemorrhagic, stellate, rapidly expanding rashes may suggest life threatening conditions (meningococcemia, septic shock, anaphylaxis, drug induced blood dyscrasias).

L. Other Care

1. History

    A thorough and concise review of the presentation and history needs to be performed. This can be most easily accomplished remembering the mnemonic "exAMPLE": **A** - allergies, **M** - medications, **P** - past illnesses, **L** - last meal, and **E** - events preceding the injury or illness.

2. Radiographic and laboratory studies .

3. Monitoring

    The patient needs to be continuously monitored and reevaluated often.

4. Consultation

    Appropriate consultants should be requested.

5. Definitive care

    The person who performs the initial evaluation and stabilization needs to remain the child's responsible physician and function as his advocate until responsibility for his total care is undertaken by another.

Chapter 2
AIRWAY MANAGEMENT

I. GOALS OF AIRWAY MANAGEMENT

A. Recognition and relief of anatomic obstruction
B. Prevention of aspiration of gastric contents
C. Promotion of adequate gas exchange

II. ANATOMY OF THE PEDIATRIC AIRWAY

The anatomic differences between infants, children, and adults are crucial to airway management (Figure 2-1).

A. **Nose**

Infants $\leq$ 6 months of age are obligate nose breathers. Anatomic or infectious obstruction will cause respiratory distress. The lymphoid tissue hemorrhages easily.

B. **Tongue**

The tongue is relatively large in relation to mandible in children < 2 years of age. Visualization of the larynx is difficult. The tongue is the most common cause of upper airway obstruction in unconscious patients of any age.

C. **Larynx**
1. Position: cervical vertebrae 2-3 in infants; cervical vertebrae 4-5 in adults (Figure 2-1).
2. Vocal cords: 40% ligament, 60% arytenoid cartilage in infants; ratios are reversed in adults.

D. **Epiglottis**
1. The **infant's** epiglottis is omega-shaped, floppy, and has a 45° angle of entry into the pharyngeal wall. Visualization of the larynx requires lifting the epiglottis directly with a straight blade.
2. The **adult's** epiglottis is stiff, flat, parallel to tracheal wall. Visualization of the larynx can be made indirectly by placing the laryngoscope blade in the vallecula (Figure 2-11).

E. **Cricoid cartilage**

Narrowest part of the airway in children < 8-10 years of age. Uncuffed endotracheal tubes are used in this age group.

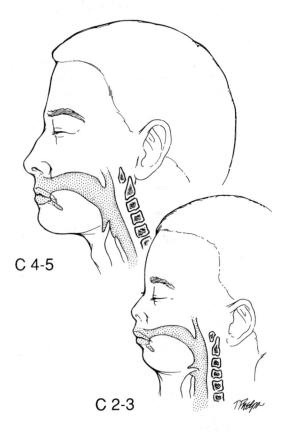

C 4-5

C 2-3

Figure 2-1. Comparative anatomy of the adult and infant airway.

TABLE 2-1. Major Causes of Upper Airway Obstruction

CNS dysfunction
- Shock
- Head trauma
- Drug overdose (alcohol, sedative/hypnotics, opioids)
- Hypoxemia/Hypercarbia
- Metabolic derangements (↑ or ↓ glucose, sodium, potassium; hepatic or uremic encephalopathy; metabolic acidosis; sepsis)
- Increased intracranial pressure leading to vocal cord paralysis (hydrocephalus, obstructed shunts)

Peripheral/Anatomic causes
- **Congenital anomalies**
  Mandibular hypoplasia:
  - *Pierre Robin* syndrome, *Treacher Collins* syndrome
  Macroglossia:
  - *Beckwith-Wiedemann* syndrome, glycogen storage diseases, hypothyroidism, *Down* syndrome
  Tracheal/laryngeal lesions:
  - Subglottic stenosis, web, cyst, laryngocele, tumor, laryngomalacia, laryngo-tracheoesophageal cleft, tracheomalacia, tracheo-esophageal fistula, juvenile papillomatosis
- **Infection**
  Supraglottic:
  - Epiglottitis, retropharyngeal abscess, Ludwig's angina, peritonsillar abscess, juvenile papillomatosis
  Subglottic:
  - Laryngotracheobronchitis (croup), staphylococcal tracheitis
- **Trauma:**
  - External trauma, post-intubation croup, post-tracheostomy removal
- **Foreign body aspiration**
- **Burns:** thermal (fire, steam), chemical (lye, acid)
- **Anaphylaxis/Laryngospasm**

III. THE COMPROMISED AIRWAY

Airway obstruction or loss of protective reflexes most commonly occurs because of depression of the central nervous system or because of peripheral/anatomic abnormalities (Table 2-1). Alternatively, the upper airway, defined as the naso-, oro-, and hypopharynx may be compromised by normal anatomic features, or anomalies, of the infant's and child's airway (Figure 2-1).

IV. ASSESSMENT

A. Patient History with Noisy Breathing and Distress

1. Does it occur with feeding (a laryngo-tracheal-esophageal cleft or fistula) or only when the child is stressed (subglottic stenosis, laryngeal web, or laryngomalacia)?

2. Is it positional? Specifically, does the prone position provide relief (a supraglottic process, epiglottitis or enlarged tongue)?

3. Is it an acute process associated with fever (croup, epiglottitis, or a retropharyngeal abscess), or with a possible foreign body aspiration, or following any trauma such as intubation?

4. Is this a chronic process associated with other problems, such as hydrocephalus (vocal cord paralysis) or neuromuscular disease (aspiration pneumonia)?

5. Will the patient eat or drink, or swallow the normal oral secretions? Dysphagia is associated with supraglottic pathology (epiglottitis or retro-pharyngeal abscess).

B. Physical Examination

While taking a history, observation and physical examination progress simultaneously (see *Chapter 1*). Signs and symptoms of upper airway obstruction include

1. Paradoxical chest movements
   a. Chest collapses inward on inspiration, abdomen protrudes outwardly.
   b. When exaggerated, the sternum "cups" inward, looking like a pectus excavatum.

2. Accessory muscle use
   a. Retractions of the intercostal and sternocleidomastoid muscles.
   b. Nasal flaring

3. Stridor
   a. Inspiratory stridor suggests obstruction above the larynx.
   b. Inspiratory <u>and</u> expiratory stridor suggest obstruction below the larynx.

4. Cough
   Brassy "croupy" cough suggests pathology below the larynx and is unusual in epiglottitis.

5. Non-specific signs of respiratory distress
   a. Decreased air movement
   b. Cyanosis/pallor
   c. Somnolence is a sign of imminent respiratory arrest.

C. Radiographic Studies
Usually unnecessary, the radiographic examination may help confirm a diagnosis suspected by history and physical examination.

1. Lateral neck film - epiglottitis, foreign body

2. Anterior-Posterior view - croup, foreign body, pneumonia, asthma
3. Fluoroscopy - foreign body, paralyzed diaphragm
4. Barium swallow - tracheal-esophageal fistula, vascular ring.

Patients suspected of having an airway problem must never be transported unattended or without a monitor to the radiology department!

V. AIRWAY EQUIPMENT

A. Nasopharyngeal airways or nasal "trumpets"

1. Indication
   Relief of nasopharyngeal obstruction. The nasal trumpet is well tolerated in conscious or semi-conscious patients, and rarely provokes vomiting or laryngospasm.

2. Insertion
   A vasoconstrictive spray such as 0.25% phenylephrine (Neosynephrine) shrinks nasal mucosa and reduces the risk of bleeding. A lubricant (2% lidocaine jelly or ointment) facilitates painless insertion.

3. Size
   Length is estimated by measuring the distance from the tip of the nose to the angle of the jaw; smaller airways can dilate a path for larger ones. Available sizes: 12-36 French.

4. Complications
   a. Epistaxis
   b. Avulsion/fracture of the adenoids or nasal conchae.

5.   Contraindications
     a.   Bleeding diathesis
     b.   Cerebrospinal fluid leak (especially with basal skull fractures because of the possibility of infection or passage of the airway into the intracranial vault);
     c.   Deformity of the nose impeding passage of the tube.

B.   Oropharyngeal Airways

1.   Indication

     a.   Relief of airway obstruction in unconscious patients.
     b.   Bite block when securing an endotracheal tube.

2.   Size

     Length is estimated by placing the airway next to the face with the flange at the level of the teeth. The tip should reach the angle of the jaw.

3.   Complications

     When placed incorrectly, it may obstruct the airway by pushing the tongue backwards into the hypopharynx.

C.   Suction

1.   Indication
     Suction of emesis, blood, particulate matter, or oral secretions.

2.   Technique
     Suction should be set at the highest vacuum rate possible.

3. Equipment
Rigid, wide bore catheters (Yankauer) or 14-18 French tracheal suction catheters.

VI. OXYGEN THERAPY EQUIPMENT

Oxygen is the first and most important drug to be used in any pediatric crisis situation. There is never a resuscitation situation in which 100% delivered oxygen is contraindicated!

Commonly used oxygen therapy equipment is depicted in Figure 2-2 and described in Table 2-2.

TABLE 2-2. Oxygen Delivery Equipment

Device	FiO$_2$	Patient Size	Comments
Nasal cannula	.22-.50	Neonate, infant, child, adult	least restrictive, best tolerated, FiO$_2$ unknown, entrains room air, does not require humidification, flows 0.5-6 L/minute
Simple face mask	.22-.50	infant, child, adult	entrains room air, requires humidification, flows 4-6 L/minute
Non-rebreathing face mask	.21-1.0	child, adult	reservoir provides 100% FiO$_2$, requires humidification, flows 4-8 L/minute
Oxygen hood	.21-1.0	neonate, infant < 10 kg	requires humidification, flows > 10 L/minute to flush out CO$_2$

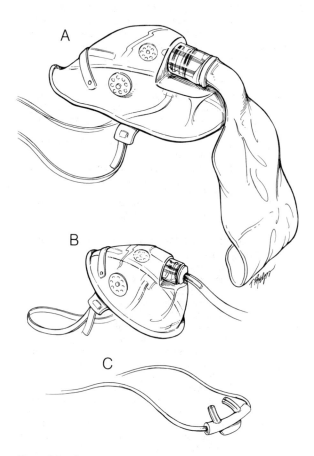

Figure 2-2. Oxygen delivery equipment. (A) Non-rebreathing face mask with reservoir. (B) Simple face mask. (C) Nasal cannula.

VII. MANUAL VENTILATION EQUIPMENT

The airway is opened with triple jaw maneuver (Figure 2-3). Once a patent airway has been established, one determines if the patient is adequately breathing. If not, manual ventilation by bag, mask, and 100% oxygen is started .

A.   Resuscitation ("Ventilation") Face Mask

1.   A face mask consists of a rubber or plastic body, a connecting port, and a rim (rigid or malleable) that allows a tight face seal during resuscitation.

2.   Equipment types

a.   Soft - with or without a cushioned edge to mold to the shape of the face.

b.   Rigid, low profile, hard edge, minimal dead space.

c.   Opaque ("black") or clear - clear masks allow early identification of emesis or excess secretions in the pharynx.

B.   Manual Resuscitation Bags or Positive Pressure Oxygen Delivery Systems

1.   Indication

The bag provides a rapid means of delivering positive pressure breaths when connected to a resuscitation face mask.

2.   Self inflating bags (Figure 2-4)

These bags entrain room air, unless a reservoir is attached for 100% O_2. Spring loaded disk valves will **not open** during spontaneous ventilation. Patients must be manually ventilated. These bags reinflate automatically after each breath.

3.   Anesthesia bags (Figure 2-5)

These require a minimum of 3 L/min flow and do not refill spontaneously. The adjustable pop-off valve requires training in its use. Patients can breathe spontaneously or can be manually ventilated. Adequacy of ventilation is easy to assess. 100% O_2 can be delivered without a reservoir.

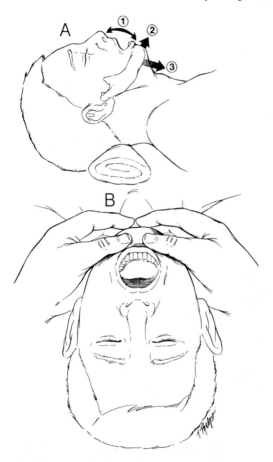

Figure 2-3. Triple jaw maneuver.
(1) Mouth open. (2) Mandible displaced anteriorly and (3) downward.

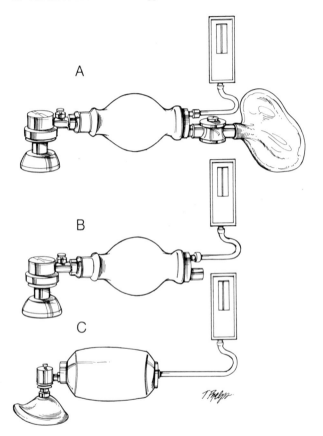

Figure 2-4. Self-inflating bags. (A) Ambu bag with reservoir for delivery of 100% oxygen. (B) Ambu bag without reservoir entrains room air. (C) PMR bag without oxygen supply valve or oxygen accumulator delivers 45 - 50% oxygen.

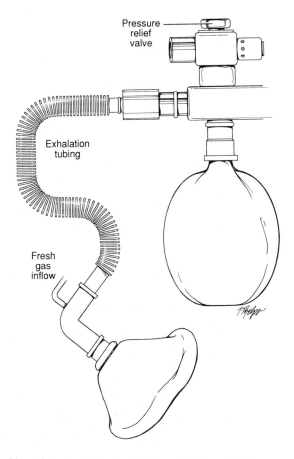

Figure 2-5. Anesthesia bag (Mapleson D delivers 100% oxygen).

VIII. BAG AND MASK VENTILATION

A. Introduction

When a patient's breathing is inadequate, the temptation is to intubate the trachea immediately. This is rarely necessary. On the other hand, ventilation and oxygenation by either mouth-to-mouth or bag and mask technique are essential and should precede intubation.

B. Bag and Mask Ventilation (Figure 2-6)

1. Adults and older children

    The mask is held in the left hand and should be pressed against the nasal bridge with the thumb at the same time that the index finger exerts downward pressure on the base of the mask over the chin. These two fingers provide the mask seal and allow the delivery of positive pressure ventilation. The middle finger lies directly on the mandible, lifting it up. The little finger engages the angle of the jaw lifting the mandible forward. The wrist is cocked to tilt the head backward.

2. Infants and small children

    As above, with the ring and little fingers floating to prevent external compression of the airway in the soft tissues of the submental area of the neck.

C. Adjuvants to Make Ventilation Easier

1. Airways

    An oro- or naso-pharyngeal airway used in conjunction with the face mask help relieve airway obstruction (usually the tongue).

2. Positive End Expiratory Pressure (PEEP)

    PEEP helps in overcoming airway obstruction by dilating the upper airway. This is helpful in spontaneously breathing patients with upper airway obstruction (epiglottitis or croup). Pressure should not exceed 15 mmHg, because it may force air into the stomach and increase the risk of vomiting and aspiration.

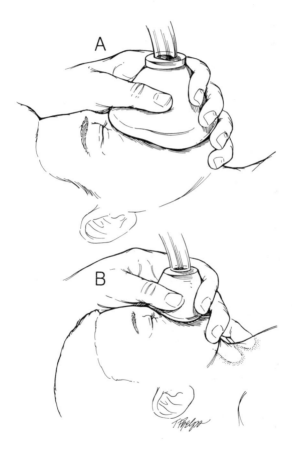

Figure 2-6. Bag and mask ventilation.

IX. INTUBATION OF THE TRACHEA

The method for intubating the trachea is dependent on:

A. Judgment of one's own intubation skills

B. Options for intubation (Table 2-3)

C. The patient's hemodynamic status

D. An assessment of the normalcy of the patient's upper airway, larynx, and trachea. Conditions associated with difficult intubation are listed in Table 2-4.

TABLE 2-3. Options for Emergency Intubation

"Awake" intubation (no sedation)
- Difficult airway: congenital anomalies; trauma; burns
- Hemodynamically unstable patient
- Unconscious patient
- Newborn

"Full stomach" precautions (Rapid pharmacologic paralysis, sedation and cricoid pressure (Figure 2-8).
- Multiple trauma, pain
- Bowel obstruction, peritonitis, peritoneal dialysis, ascites
- History of gastroesophageal reflux (history of gastroesophageal fistula repair)
- Pregnancy (> 2nd trimester)
- Increased intracranial pressure
- Undocumented fasting period or documented fast of < 8 hours for solid food.

General anesthesia requires operating room, anesthesiologist and surgeon for possible bronchoscopy and tracheostomy.
- Airway obstruction (acute supraglottitis)
- Foreign body aspiration

Sedation and paralysis
- Elective intubation (prior to gastric lavage, radiographic procedures, cardioversion)

TABLE 2-4. Syndromes Associated with Difficult Intubation

- Micrognathia:
  Cri-du-chat (also narrow larynx); *DiGeorge* syndrome (also hypocalcemic tetany); *Pierre Robin* syndrome; *Treacher Collins* syndrome; *Noonan* syndrome; *Turner* syndrome; Trisomy 13, 18
- Macroglossia:
  Beckwith-Wiedemann syndrome; Trisomy 21 (*Down* syndrome); *Hurler* and *Hunter* syndrome (mucopolysaccharidoses) (also short neck); Hypothyroidism; Glycogen storage disease (*Pompe* disease); *Scheie* syndrome (prognathism, short neck)
- Midface hypoplasia; Craniofacial dysostosis (maxilla and/or mandible):
  Apert syndrome; *Crouzon* syndrome; *Goldenhar* syndrome (oculo-auriculo-vertebral); Median cleft face syndrome (cleft lip, nose, palate); Cherubism (fibrous dysplasia of mandible); hemi-facial microsomia
- Short neck - rigid neck:
  Ankylosing spondylitis; Rheumatoid arthritis; *Hurler* syndrome; *Hunter* syndrome; *Morquio* syndrome; *Klippel-Feil* syndrome
- Temporomandibular joint diseases:
  Collagen vascular diseases (rheumatoid arthritis, polyarteritis nodosa, dermatomyositis, systemic lupus erythematosus); Trismus (following trauma, local infection); Infection (*Ludwig* angina, retropharyngeal abscess); Arthrogryposis multiplex
- Airway edema/fibrosis:
  Angioedema (anaphylaxis, hereditary); Pregnancy; Epidermolysis Bullosa; *Stevens-Johnson* syndrome;
- Any patient in a halo traction device

X. DRUGS FOR INTUBATION

A. Neuromuscular Blocking Agents (Table 2-5)

These drugs are classified by:
1. Mechanism
   a. Depolarizing muscle relaxants (succinylcholine)
   b. Non-depolarizing muscle relaxants (pancuronium, vecuronium, atracurium, d-tubocurarine)
2. Duration of action:
   a. Short (succinylcholine)
   b. Intermediate (vecuronium, atracurium)
   c. Long (pancuronium, d-tubocurarine)

B. Antagonism of Neuromuscular Blockade

Non-depolarizing muscle relaxants act by competitive inhibition of the neuromuscular junction and can be antagonized ("reversed") with acetylcholinesterase inhibitors. Circumstances that prevent adequate antagonism include: intense blockade, respiratory acidosis, drug interactions (aminoglycosides), organ failure (liver, kidney), hypothermia.

C. Sedative/Hypnotics and Analgesics (Table 2-6)

It is intolerable to paralyze an awake patient! The proper agent and dose are dependent on the patient's clinical condition and hemodynamic status. It must be emphasized that there are no "correct" dosages of these drugs. Some patients may require enormous amounts of drug and others very little. The only way to use these drugs is by titration to effect. It is always better to use the lower dosages and to titrate upward as needed. Suggested doses are listed in Table 2-6.

TABLE 2-5. Neuromuscular Blocking Agents

Drug	Contraindications	Side effects, comments
Succinylcholine Dose: IV 1-2 mg/kg IM 3-4 mg/kg Onset: IV 30-60 sec. IM 180 sec Duration: IV 3-10 min IM 5-20 min	Myasthenia gravis; *Guillain-Barre* syndrome; demyelinating disease; crush-, burn-, electrical-injuries, spinal cord injuries after 24 hrs; open globe injury; malignant hyperthermia; myotonia congenita; ↑ intracranial pressure	1. Dysrhythmias: sinus arrest, bradycardia, nodal and ventricular arrhythmias. 2. Fasciculations: ↑ intra -abdominal,-thoracic, and -cranial pressure. 3. Muscle pain: 10% of patients, ↓ pain with prior defasciculation using 0.01 mg/kg pancuronium. 4. Potassium efflux (↑ serum [K⁺] 0.5 meq/L in all patients); [K⁺] ≥ 10 mEq/L in myasthenia, *Guillain-Barre* syndrome, spinal cord injury (starts 24 hours after injury and lasts for 6 months), crush or electrical injury. 6. Contraction of extraocular muscles. 7. Muscle rigidity: myotonic dystrophy, malignant hyperthermia. 8. Non-reversible, requires plasma cholinesterase for biodegradation

Drug	Contraindications	Side effects, comments
Pancuronium Dose: 0.1-0.2 mg/kg Onset: 120 sec Duration: 45-90 min	Renal failure. Tricyclic antidepressant use	1. Vagolytic: ↑ heart rate and blood pressure. 2. 60-90% renal elimination. 3. Reversible in ~ 45-60 min after IV dose. 4. Interaction with tricyclic antidepressants → ventricular arrhythmias.
Vecuronium Dose: 0.1-0.2 mg/kg Onset: 45-120 sec Duration: 30-90 min	none	1. No effect on heart rate or blood pressure. 2. < 25% renal elimination. 3. Reversible in ~ 30-45 min after IV dose.
Curare Dose: 0.6 mg/kg Onset: 240-420 sec Duration: 45-90 min	Asthma, hypotension, need for rapid onset	1. Histamine release. 2. Very slow onset even at ↑ dose 3. 40-60% renal excretion 4. Reversible in ~ 45-60 min after IV dose.
Atracurium Dose: 0.4-0.7mg/kg Onset: 240-420 sec Duration: 30-45 min	Asthma, hypotension, need for rapid onset	1. Histamine release. 2. Very slow onset even at ↑ dose. 3. Hoffman elimination and ester hydrolysis, makes it ideal for kidney or liver failure patients. 4. Reversible in ~ 30-45 min after IV dose.

Drug	Contraindications	Side effects, comments
Neostigmine Dose: 0.07 mg/kg, max 3.0 mg Onset: 180-600 sec Duration: 75 min + **Atropine** Dose: 0.01 mg/kg Onset: 15-30 sec Duration: 90 min		Used to antagonize non-depolarizing neuromuscular blockade. Muscarinic effects: bradycardia, salivation, bladder contraction, bronchospasm. **Must always pretreat with atropine.**

TABLE 2-6. Intravenous Sedatives, Hypnotics, and Opioids for Intubation

Drug	Dosage (mg/kg)	Indications and Comments
Thiopental or Thiamylal in: •Normovolemia •Hypovolemia	4-7 0.25-1	•Produces general anesthesia, amnesia rapidly (< 30 sec); anti-convulsant •↓ ICP; ↓ cerebral blood flow (CBF), ↓ cerebral oxygen consumption ($CMRO_2$); no analgesic properties •Myocardial depression; hypotension in hypovolemia; apnea, respiratory depression; intraarterial injections → gangrene because pH > 11
Methohexital in: •Normovolemia **Methohexital** (rectal admin.)	1-2 30	•As above; hiccoughing, myoclonic jerking •Given rectally is useful for imaging studies (60-90 min of sedation)
Ketamine in: •Normovolemia •Hypovolemia •Intramuscular	1-2 0.5 3-7	•Potent analgesic (2 X more potent than morphine), amnestic, hallucinogen •Rapid loss of consciousness (< 30 sec) •Bronchodilator, ideal for asthmatics; ↑ oral secretions, requires anti-sialogogue (atropine); blunts airway protective reflexes •Emergence delirium and nightmares which may be prevented with concomitant benzodiazepine •Contraindicated with ↑ ICP because of ↑ cerebral blood flow •Useful in Congenital Heart Disease except Aortic Stenosis

Drug	Dosage (mg/kg)	Indications and Comments
Etomidate	0.2	• Rapid loss of consciousness (< 1 min) • Virtually no hemodynamic effects • Blunts steroidogenesis with prolonged use • Painful on IV injection, pretreat with fentanyl (0.002mg/kg) • Myoclonic jerks common; anti-convulsant, ↓ ICP, CBF, $CMRO_2$
Midazolam in • Normovolemia IM Rectally • Hypovolemia	0.2-0.3 0.1-.15 0.5-1 0.05-0.1	• Sedative/anxiolytic; general anesthetic at higher doses; amnestic, no analgesic properties; anti-convulsant • Minimal hemodynamic effects • Apnea following rapid IV administration • ↓ ICP, CBF, $CMRO_2$
Fentanyl	0.002-0.01	• Potent analgesic blunts response to intubation; mildly sedating • Hemodynamically most stable of all opioids • Chest wall rigidity at high (>0.005 mg/kg) dose, reversed with either naloxone or succinylcholine (or pancuronium)
Lidocaine	1-2	• Analgesic, decreases the cardiovascular responses to intubation when administered either intravenously or topically (4% solution) • ↓ ICP spikes associated with intubation and respiratory toilet
Scopolamine	0.02	• Amnestic, antisialogogue • Can be administered intravenously or intramuscularly • Mild tachycardia, no blood pressure effects

XI. INTUBATION EQUIPMENT

A. Laryngoscope

1. Handles

Different handle shapes and sizes are available. Pick one that fits most securely in your hand.

2. Blades (Table 2-7, 2-8, Figure 2-7):

a. Miller (straight), size 0-4: infants-adults

b. MacIntosh (curved), size 1-4: children-adult

3. Light Failure

The electrical contact between the handle and blade and between the bulb and its socket commonly corrode and prevent the flow of electricity. This can usually be scraped clean. Always be prepared for equipment failure by having extra handles and blades available.

B. Endotracheal Tubes

1. Equipment types

a. Uncuffed endotracheal tubes

Patients less than 8-10 years of age receive uncuffed endotracheal tubes to reduce the risk of subglottic edema and stenosis. An uncuffed tube of appropriate size will provide a reasonable seal at the cricoid ring, the narrowest part of the airway.

b. Cuffed endotracheal tubes

In children > 10 years, the cuff should not be inflated above 25 mmHg pressure or mucosal ischemia or necrosis may occur.

2. Size (Table 2-7, 2-8)

The internal diameter of the endotracheal tube can be estimated by using the formula:

$$(16 + \text{age in years})/4$$

Always have additional tubes available, one size smaller and one size larger than the calculated size.

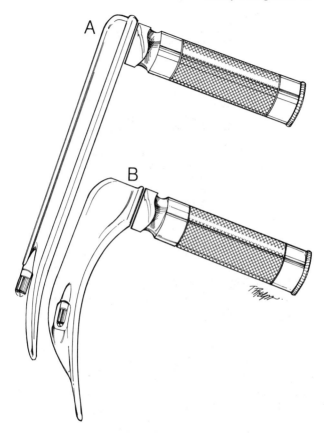

Figure 2-7. Laryngoscope Blades. (A) Straight (Miller).
(B) Curved (MacIntosh)

C. Stylets

1. Definition

    Elongated metal or plastic rod that alters the natural curve of an endotracheal tube and facilitates intubation.

2. Indication

    When difficult intubation is anticipated.

3. Technique

    a. Lubricate the stylet before inserting it to facilitate its removal after intubation.

    b. The stylet must never extend beyond the distal end of the endotracheal tube and it must never be used to force entry into the trachea!

4. Complications

    a. Submucosal dissection

    b. Lacerations, hemorrhage, hematomas

    c. Tracheal perforation

    d. Pneumothorax

    e. Pneumomediastinum

TABLE 2-7. Intubation Equipment Sizes

Age (years)	Laryngoscope blade (size)	ID (mm)	Length (cm) Oral	Suction
Premature	0	2.5-3.0	7-9	5 Fr
Newborn	0	3.5	9-11	6 Fr
1	1	4.0	12	8 Fr
2	2	4.5	13	10 Fr
4	2	5.0	14	10 Fr
6	2	5.5	15	10 Fr
8	2-3	6.0	16	10 Fr

TABLE 2-8. Intubation Equipment Checklist

Suction:
- Large bore, disposable tracheal suction catheters (14-18 F); Yankauer "tonsil sucker"

Oxygen delivery equipment:
- Bag-valve ventilation device (Ambu bag, Laerdal bag, Vital Signs disposable bag)
- Anesthesia ventilation bag (Mapleson C, D)

Airway:
- Oro-pharyngeal airways, various sizes
- Naso-pharyngeal airways, various sizes

Face masks:
- Various sizes (Rendell-Baker, Vital-Signs, Ohio)

Laryngoscope blades:
- Miller "straight" blades, sizes: 0, 1, 1.5, 2, 3, 4
- MacIntosh "curved" blades, sizes: 2, 3, 4

Endotracheal tubes:
- Uncuffed 2.5-7 mm ID, up to 8-10 years of age
- Cuffed 5-9 mm ID, 8 years of age and older

Stylet and lubricant
Tongue depressor
Adhesive tape and skin protector
(tincture of benzoin, mastisol)

Monitoring equipment:
- Pulse oximeter
- ECG
- Blood pressure cuff

Drugs:
- Atropine
- Muscle relaxant
- Sedative

XII. TECHNIQUES FOR INTUBATION

A. Preoxygenation
Ventilation with 100% O_2 should always precede intubation to avoid prolonged hypoxia.

B. Monitoring
ECG, pulse oximetry, and noninvasive blood pressure are the minimum requirements, except during cardiorespiratory arrest when immediate intubation is necessary.

C. Equipment Preparation
Table 2-8 is a checklist of essential equipment necessary for intubation that must be reviewed prior to intubation.

D. Positioning
Successful intubation requires proper positioning of the head and neck, opening the mouth widely, proper insertion of laryngoscope with clear visualization of the vocal cords and proper placement of the endotracheal tube (Figure 2-9, 2-10).

1. Head and neck
    The proper position for the head and neck maximizes the alignment of the laryngeal axis with the oropharyngeal axis and mouth. The head is tilted backwards, extending the atlanto-occipital joint with the hand and by elevating the occiput with a folded towel underneath the head ("sniffing" position). Extension of the head without elevation of the occiput rotates the larynx anteriorly and makes visualization difficult.

2. Cervical Spine Injury
    Patients with cervical spine injury require special consideration. An assistant straddles the patient and places his/her hands on the patient's mastoid processes. A gentle traction force in the cephalad direction is applied, keeping the mastoid process in

line. This should counter any extension or flexion of the cervical spine during laryngoscopy.

E. Opening the Mouth

The mouth is opened widely by depressing the lower teeth and mandible with the right thumb while pushing against the upper teeth with the right middle finger ("scissor maneuver").   This minimizes trauma to the teeth, lips and gums.

F. Cricoid Pressure (Figure 2-8)

Compression of the cricoid ring with the thumb and index finger occludes the esophagus and prevents passive regurgitation. It may also help visualize the larynx. In rapid sequence intubation cricoid pressure is maintained until tube placement is confirmed.

G. Laryngoscopy

1.   Blade Insertion

The laryngoscope blade is gripped firmly in the left hand and inserted from the right side of the mouth, gently lifting and sweeping the tongue to the left (Figure 2-9). The visualized larynx is seen in Figure 2-10.

2.   Curved Blade Advancement (Figure 2-11)

The curved blade is advanced slowly along the base of the tongue until the epiglottis is visualized. The tip of the blade is inserted into the space between the base of the tongue and the epiglottis (the vallecula). The operator's wrist is then fixed in position and further exposure gained by lifting the laryngoscope vertically forward without using leverage on maxillary structures. The epiglottis is elevated and the glottis visualized. Pressure on the thyroid cartilage may improve visualization of the glottis. Never pull backwards, or flex your wrist, or lean on the upper teeth with the laryngoscope blade.

3. Straight Blade Advancement (Figure 2-11)
The straight blade is advanced below the epiglottis along the posterior wall. The laryngoscope is then lifted and retracted slowly while elevating the soft tissue until the glottis appears. The endotracheal tube is placed as above. The straight blade is the preferred blade in children because the epiglottis is so floppy. Inserting the curved or straight blade into the vallecula may result in failure because the vertical lift of the blade may not pull up the epiglottis (Figure 2-11).

H. Placement of the Endotracheal Tube

The tube is inserted from the right side, using a stylet if necessary, and the tip passed between the vocal cords.

1. Uncuffed endotracheal tube
The distal line markings should be used to gauge the depth of insertion. If the endotracheal tube has a single distal line marker, that line should be visible at the true vocal cords. If the endotracheal tube has two or three distal line markers, the second or third line markers should be visible above the true vocal cords.

2. Cuffed endotracheal tube
Advancement of the tube should stop as soon as the cuff is below the vocal cords. Failure to do this often results in endobronchial intubation.

I. Endotracheal Tube Position Confirmation

Endotracheal tube position must be confirmed and the tube must be stabilized and secured with waterproof adhesives (Table 2-9).

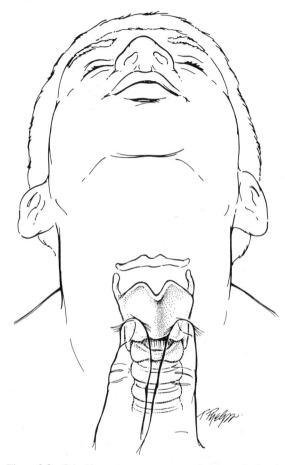

Figure 2-8. Cricoid pressure to prevent passive regurgitation during intubation.

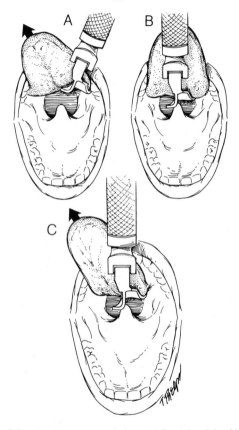

Figure 2-9. The laryngoscope is inserted from the right side of the mouth. The tongue is swept from the right to the left.
(A) INCORRECT- The laryngoscope has not returned to the middle.
(B) INCORRECT- The tongue hangs over the right side of the blade.
(C) CORRECT- Final position.

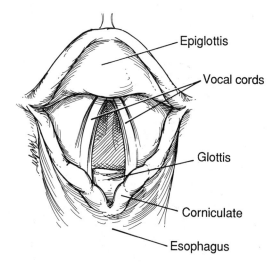

Figure 2-10. Larynx.

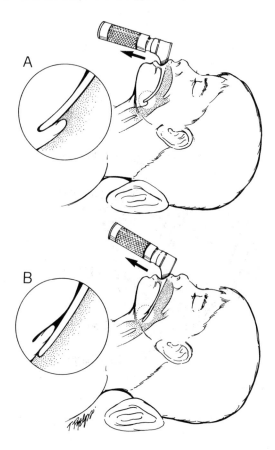

Figure 2-11. Sagittal view of laryngoscopy.
(A) Curved blade is placed in the vallecula;
(B) The tip of straight blade is placed under the epiglottis.

TABLE 2-9.   **Endotracheal Tube Position Confirmation and Stabilization**

Visual inspection

- Laryngoscopy (tube through the cords, no visible cuff, distal line marker visible at the level of the vocal cords)
- Symmetrical chest wall movement with ventilation
- The epigastrium does not bulge with ventilation
- Inflation of the reservoir bag (anesthesia type bag) with each exhalation

Auscultation

- Breath sounds in both lung fields, preferably in the axilla
- No low pitched gurgling in the stomach

Mechanical

- Carbon dioxide tension in end-tidal gas (most reliable, rarely available)
- Chest X-ray (tip of the tube in mid trachea)
- Pulse oximetry (oxygenation should improve)

Stabilization

- Bite block (oral airway)
- Skin adhesive (tincture of benzoin, mastisol)
- Waterproof tape (secured to the maxilla)

XIII. COMPLICATIONS OF INTUBATION

A. Complications During Laryngoscopy or Intubation

1. Corneal abrasion
2. Dental and soft tissue trauma (laceration, abrasion, tooth loss)
3. Cardiac dysrhythmia
4. Autonomic instability
   a. Hypertension, tachycardia
   b. Hypotension, bradycardia
   c. Vagally mediated reflexes (apnea, laryngospasm, bronchospasm, vomiting)
5. Aspiration of stomach contents
6. Esophageal intubation
7. Endobronchial intubation
8. Arytenoid cartilage dislocation

B. Complications with the Tube in Place

1. Increased resistance to breathing
2. Endotracheal tube obstruction ("plugging")
3. Accidental extubation
4. Autonomic instability (see above)

C. Complications After Intubation

1. Laryngeal damage or edema (pharyngitis, laryngitis, laryngeal granuloma or ulceration, laryngeal web, vocal cord paralysis)
2. Tracheal damage or edema (tracheal mucosa ischemia, tracheal stenosis)

XIV.   CRICOTHYROTOMY (Figure 2-12)

A.   Indications

Occasionally, a patient can neither be ventilated nor intubated and an emergency needle cricothyrotomy is required to establish the airway.

B.   Technique

When performing an emergency cricothyrotomy, the neck is extended and the thyroid and cricoid cartilages identified. The skin is cleaned with antiseptic. A number 14 gauge, 5 cm catheter-over-the-needle apparatus is attached to a 5 cc syringe. The needle is directed at a 45° angle caudally in the midline of the cricothyroid membrane. The syringe is aspirated while advancing the needle until air is obtained. The catheter is advanced over the needle and an endotracheal tube adapter from a 3.0 mm (pediatric) endotracheal tube is inserted into the hub of the catheter. The catheter is secured and the endotracheal tube adaptor is connected to a positive pressure ventilation bag to allow ventilation with 100% O_2. The chest is then observed and auscultated to assess the adequacy of ventilation. This is a temporary measure only and alternative methods for securing the airway should be undertaken. Complications of needle cricothyrotomy include hemorrhage, aspiration, asphyxia, perforation of trachea and esophagus, and pneumothorax.

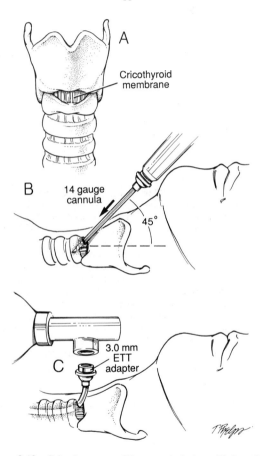

Figure 2-12. Cricothyrotomy. (A) anatomical view. (B) Insertion of 14 gauge IV cannula. (C) Bag attached to 3.0 endotracheal tube (ETT) adaptor connected to IV cannula.

Chapter 3
EPIGLOTTITIS AND CROUP

I. OVERVIEW

Croup and epiglottitis are the most frequent causes of life-threatening acute upper airway obstruction in early childhood. Patients with these infections may suffer unexpected respiratory arrests, if the severity of illness and airway obstruction is not appreciated. A successful outcome is dependent on rapid, accurate diagnosis, an appreciation of the severity of the obstruction, and the appropriate management by a skilled medical team.

A. Pathophysiology

The laws of physics (Poiseuille's and Bernoulli's Laws) that govern the flow of gas through narrow tubes explain the susceptibility of infants and small children to acute upper airway obstruction. The clinical presentation with respiratory distress, retractions and stridor is frequently more dramatic in small children than in adults.

TABLE 3-1. Poiseuille's Law

Laminar Flow: $\text{Resistance} = \dfrac{K \times \text{viscosity}}{\text{radius}^4}$

Turbulent Flow: $\text{Resistance} = \dfrac{K \times \text{density}}{\text{radius}^5}$

---

1. Poiseuille's Law (Table 3-1)

    With turbulent gas flow (as occurs with air flow through a narrowing of a large conducting airway) the resistance to breathing is inversely proportional to the radius[5], i.e., the resistance will increase 32 times if the airway is narrowed by half its diameter. Such a reduction is easily accomplished by relatively minor edema of the narrow airway of an infant, compared with the same amount of edema in the wider airway of an adult (Figure 3-1). With severe airway obstruction, the diameter of the airway lumen may be reduced by an even greater extent providing a correspondingly greater resistance to breathing.

2. Bernoulli's Principle (Figure 3-2)

    In addition to the pathologic process (e.g., epiglottitis or viral croup) that produces the fixed airway obstruction, Bernoulli's principle (Table 3-2) accounts for a dynamic obstruction that is superimposed upon the collapsible extrathoracic airway. This phenomenon is caused by the acceleration of air flow across the site of the fixed obstruction and is manifested as worsening of stridor and respiratory distress during agitation and crying.

TABLE 3-2. Bernoulli's Principle

When gas flows through a narrowing in a collapsible tube, the pressure that holds the tube open will decrease (thereby causing collapse of the tube) as the velocity of flow through the constriction increases.

B. A General Approach to the Child with Acute Upper Airway Obstruction.

Acute upper airway obstruction is suggested by the clinical features of respiratory distress with stridor, retraction, tachypnea and even cyanosis. The following sequential steps should be adopted when faced with a child with upper airway obstruction regardless of the etiology (Table 3-3).

TABLE 3-3.   General Clinical Approach to the Child with Acute Upper Airway Obstruction

---

Determine the severity of obstruction

- Stridor, retractions, air entry, color, consciousness

- Is therapeutic intervention necessary prior to precise diagnosis?

Determine the etiology of obstruction

- History, physical examination: prodrome, rate of progression, sore throat, drooling, voice, fever

- Radiology (x-ray neck, chest)

- Endoscopy

- Other laboratory tests (CBC, cultures)

Careful monitoring for respiratory deterioration

Initiate supportive and specific therapy

CROSS SECTION OF INFANT'S TRACHEA
AT THE CRICOID CARTILAGE

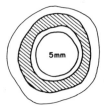

DEVELOPMENT
OF SUBMUCOSAL
EDEMA

Figure 3-1. Marked reduction in the caliber of the airway lumen of an infant compared with that of an adult when caused by only a mild degree of submucosal edema.

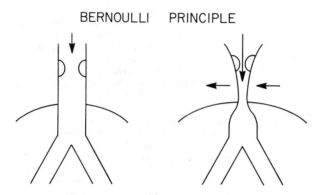

Figure 3-2. Dynamic obstruction superimposed upon the collapsible extrathoracic airway by acceleration of air flow across the site of narrowing.

1. Determine the severity of airway obstruction.

   a. Assess primarily on the basis of clinical findings the degree of stridor, color, retractions, air entry and level of consciousness (Table 3-4). This scale was devised to evaluate the severity of respiratory distress in children with laryngotracheobronchitis.

   b. Arterial puncture for blood gas determination can worsen obstruction by increasing the patient's agitation and should be avoided in most cases.

   c. Decide whether urgent establishment of an artificial airway with endotracheal intubation is indicated (*Chapter 2*).

2. Determine the etiology of obstruction.

   If the child is stable, an abbreviated history, physical examination and further workup can be completed to determine a precise diagnosis. The history should include details of a prodrome, the rate of progression of symptoms, the presence of a fever, sore throat, dysphagia, drooling, changes in phonation, and foreign body aspiration.

3. Clinical observation and monitoring to detect deterioration.

   The child must be closely observed and monitored so that deterioration from worsening airway obstruction will be noticed.

4. Specific therapy.

   Once a specific diagnosis has been made, appropriate therapy can be implemented such as intubation, tracheostomy, drug therapy to decrease airway edema, antibiotics, etc.

TABLE 3-4. Estimation of Severity of Respiratory Distress

DEGREE OF SEVERITY

SIGN	0	1	2	3
Stridor	none	only with agitation	mild at rest	severe at rest
Retraction	none	mild	moderate	severe at rest
Air entry	normal	mild ↓	moderate ↓	marked ↓
Color	normal	normal	normal	cyanotic
Level of consciousness	normal	restless when disturbed	restless when undisturbed	lethargic

From: Fleisher GR: Infectious Disease Emergencies, in Fleisher GR, Ludwig S, eds. **Textbook of Pediatric Emergency Medicine**, Williams and Wilkins, 1986. Reproduced with permission.

C. Differential Diagnosis

The differential diagnosis of acute upper airway obstruction is outlined in Table 3-5 (also see Table 2-1) but only those entities causing acute airway obstruction with fever are emphasized.

TABLE 3-5.	Differential Diagnosis of Acute Upper Airway Obstruction

- Viral laryngotracheobronchitis[*]
- Spasmodic croup
- Epiglottitis
- Retropharyngeal abscess
- Bacterial tracheitis
- Peritonsillar abscess
- Foreign body aspiration
- Corrosive ingestion
- Neck trauma
- Angioedema
- Diphtheria
- Infectious mononucleosis

[*]Recurrent Croup may indicate an anatomic airway abnormality, e.g., subglottic stenosis or hemangioma.

II. LARYNGOTRACHEOBRONCHITIS

Laryngotracheobronchitis has been divided into 3 categories - viral laryngotracheobronchitis (croup), spasmodic croup, and bacterial tracheitis which must be distinguished from epiglottitis and retropharyngeal abscess (Table 3-6).

A. Classification

1. Viral Laryngotracheobronchitis (LTB)

Viral Laryngotracheobronchitis is usually caused by the parainfluenza virus types 1 and 2 or by the respiratory syncytial virus. Upper respiratory infection (URI) symptoms develop followed by a "barking" cough, stridor, and respiratory distress. Symptoms vary over several days with stridor usually worsening at night. Most patients require minimal or no treatment, but up to 10% of affected children require hospitalization, and <5% of hospitalized patients require an artificial airway to relieve obstruction.

TABLE 3-6. Diagnostic Features of Infectious Causes of Stridor

	Viral croup	Epiglottitis	Bacterial Tracheitis	Retropharyngeal Abscess
History: Age	2 mo - 4 yr	3-6 yr (up to adult)	2-4 yr	children-adults
Prodrome	None or URI	None	URI	Pharyngitis, trauma
Onset	Gradual	Fulminant	Variable	Slow
Dysphagia	±	+++	±	+++
Signs: Fever	Low grade	High, toxic	High, toxic	Variable
Stridor	+++	++	+++	+
Drooling	−	+++	±	+++
Posture	Lying	Sitting	Variable	Variable
Tests: WBC	<10,000	>10,000	>10,000	>10,000
x-ray	Subglottic narrowing	Swollen supraglottis	Subglottic irregularity	Widened retropharynx
Cultures	Parainfluenza, RSV	H. flu, Strep	S. aureus	Staph, Strep, Anaerobes

2. Spasmodic Croup

    Spasmodic Croup is a distinct entity usually characterized by recurrent episodes of acute stridor with or without a febrile URI prodrome. The onset of clinical symptoms is usually acute and at night and the course is usually mild. Resolution frequently occurs with emesis or exposure to cold air or mist. Both forms of croup occur in children of similar ages and with similar associated viral pathogens. It has been suggested that spasmodic croup may be an allergic reaction to viral antigens rather than a true infection.

3. Bacterial Tracheitis

    Bacterial tracheitis is an uncommon infection usually caused by a secondary staphylococcus aureus infection superimposed upon viral laryngotracheobronchitis. This infection is characterized by infraglottic inflammation with extensive exudate and edema within the trachea and bronchi. Affected children usually become acutely ill and toxic after a prodromal viral illness and develop respiratory distress and stridor. The diagnosis is frequently made after endoscopic examination of the airway which is performed because of worsening respiratory distress or the clinical suspicion of epiglottitis.

B. Management

1. General Approach

    In the emergency room, therapy and triage can be instituted once a correct diagnosis has been made, the severity of disease assessed, and close monitoring to detect clinical deterioration is operative. The intensity of care is adjusted as the child's condition changes (Table 3-7).

TABLE 3-7.	Hospital Therapy of Viral Laryngotracheobronchitis	

Croup Score (Table 3-4)	Clinical Severity	Management
≤ 4	mild	Outpatient mist therapy
5-6	mild - moderate	Outpatient if: (1) child improves in ER after mist, (2) is >6 months old, and (3) has reliable parents
7-8	moderate	Admit, give racemic epinephrine
≥ 9	severe	Admit to ICU, racemic epinephrine, possible intubation

From: Fleisher GR: Infectious Disease Emergencies, in Fleisher GR, Ludwig S, eds. **Textbook of Pediatric Emergency Medicine**, Williams and Wilkins, 1986. Reproduced with permission.

2. Specific Measures
   a. Minimal disturbance. Avoid agitation such as obtaining blood gases in all but the most severe cases. Usually, severity can be judged clinically (Table 3-4).
   b. Humidified Oxygen.
   c. Fever control, hydration if necessary.
   d. **Racemic epinephrine**. The efficacy of this drug is based on the alpha adrenergic properties of epinephrine that produce topical mucosal vasoconstriction thereby reducing mucosal edema.

Dose: 0.05 ml/kg of 2.25% solution diluted with 3 ml normal saline.

Maximum dose: 0.5 ml (of 2.25% solution).

Interval: May be used as frequently as q 30 min if patient is monitored to avoid severe tachycardia. **If no improvement after 3 doses in 90 min., consider intubation.**

Administer by nebulization rather than intermittent positive pressure breathing which is better tolerated, easier to administer, and has less risk of barotrauma.

e.   Patients receiving racemic epinephrine should be admitted to the hospital because of the potential for rebound worsening of airway obstruction.

f.   Corticosteroids

A recent study suggests that dexamethasone 0.6 mg/kg is effective in reducing the severity of moderate to severe disease. (Super DM et al, J Pediatr 115: 323-329, 1989).

g.   Antibiotics

There is no need for antibiotic therapy in viral laryngotracheobronchitis once epiglottitis, bacterial tracheitis, or retropharyngeal abscess have been ruled out.

h.   Airway management

Helium/oxygen mixture.

Because of its low density, helium reduces the work of breathing by decreasing the resistance to turbulent gas flow through a narrowed airway (Poiseuille's law).   It should only be used in an intensive care unit with continuous pulse oximetry monitoring to avoid hypoxia.   At least 70% helium must be used to be effective.

Establishment of an artificial airway (endotracheal intubation/tracheotomy) is mandatory for the management of respiratory failure secondary to upper airway obstruction (see Table 4-11 for techniques). Table 3-8 outlines the indications for intubation of a patient with viral croup.

TABLE 3-8. **Indications for Intubation of a Patient with Viral Laryngotracheobronchitis**

- increasing severity of retractions
- decreasing air entry
- worsening stridor
- decreased stridor but increased expiratory wheeze
- cyanosis
- depressed sensorium
- worsening hypoxia and/or hypercarbia

III. EPIGLOTTITIS

A. Clinical Manifestations

Epiglottitis, or more appropriately supraglottitis, is characterized by bacterial infection of the supraglottis (epiglottis, arytenoids, aryepiglottic folds), usually with sparing of the subglottic areas. *Haemophilus influenzae* type b (*H flu*) is the predominant bacterial pathogen. This disease tends to occur in toddlers and young children but may be seen in infants and adults. The typical clinical picture is characterized by acute onset of high fever, sore throat, dysphagia, and drooling. Vocal and respiratory changes such as muffled voice, reluctance to speak and stridor without cough are typical. Patients are reluctant to lie supine because this posture aggravates airway obstruction, and they frequently sit in a tripod fashion with head extended and mouth open. Patients may develop complete airway obstruction within a few hours of the onset of symptoms.

B. Management

When the diagnosis of epiglottitis is suspected by the examining physician in the emergency room, the following steps should be instituted:

1. Minimal disturbance.
   Avoid procedures that may precipitate sudden airway obstruction.
   a. Do not examine pharynx with tongue blade.
   b. Allow the child to sit up in parent's lap.
   c. Do not place supine.
   d. Do not draw blood, place IV, or obtain cultures. This will be performed in the operating room.

2. Oxygen.
   Provide oxygen by face mask if tolerated by the child.

3. Airway management.
   Activate "epiglottitis protocol." Every hospital should have an epiglottitis protocol that defines a multi-disciplinary team (pediatrician, anesthesiologist, otolaryngologist or surgeon) that can evaluate and secure the airway in the child with epiglottitis. The diagnostic and therapeutic steps in the emergency room will depend upon the severity of the illness as judged by the emergency room physicians.
   a. If the patient is unstable with upper airway obstruction (unresponsive, cyanotic, or with bradycardia) then,
      (1) ventilate with bag and mask and 100% oxygen (*Chapter 2*).

       (2)   perform emergency laryngoscopy and intubation by the most skilled individual available.

    b.   If the diagnosis is questionable and the patient is stable, then an attempt should be made to confirm the diagnosis with the lateral neck x-ray (Figure 3-3). Individuals skilled in airway management must remain with the child at all times.

    c.   If epiglottitis is highly suspected or confirmed by x-ray, the child should be transported to the operating room for upper airway endoscopy and intubation under general anesthesia. Transportation is a high risk procedure. The child must be accompanied by a physician skilled in airway management and with parents present to pacify the child.

       (1)   Monitoring en route to the OR should consist of ECG and pulse oximetry if possible.

       (2)   Oxygen should be administered by face mask if tolerated.

       (3)   Bag, mask, laryngoscope, blades, endotracheal tubes (include smaller sizes), stylets, 14 gauge angiocath for transtracheal ventilation and emergency drugs should accompany the child.

4.   Intensive Care Management of Epiglottitis

Once the airway has been secured in the operating room by endotracheal intubation, the child should be transported to an intensive care unit.

    a.   Monitoring includes ECG, blood pressure, O_2 saturation.

    b.   Frequent suctioning of endotracheal tube to prevent plugging.

c. Arm restraints and sedation (valium, midazolam, morphine) to prevent agitation and accidental extubation.

d. Be alert for the development of pulmonary edema.

e. Be alert for the development of other foci of infection (e.g., pneumonia and meningitis).

f. IV antibiotics: e.g., ceftriaxone (75 mg/kg/day divided q 12h), cefotaxime (100 mg/kg/day divided q 6h). Add oxacillin if bacterial tracheitis is diagnosed at endoscopy.

g. If the etiology is *H. flu* and at least 1 household member is less than 48 months of age, then rifampin prophylaxis for all household contacts including index case is administered: < 1 month: 10/mg/kg/day q.d. X 4 days; > 1 month: 20 mg/kg/day q.d. X 4 days; max dose 600 mg/day.

h. Extubate when:
   (1) Fever has responded to antibiotic therapy (need not be afebrile).
   (2) Leak around endotracheal tube is less than 25 cm of water.
   (3) Epiglottic inflammation and swelling have resolved (nasopharyngoscopy or laryngoscopy with IV sedation).
   (4) Usual duration of intubation is 24-48 hours.

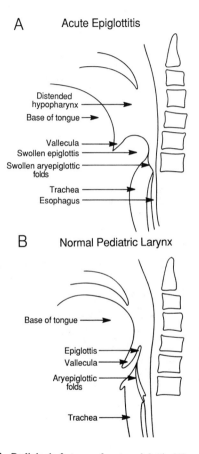

Figure 3-3. Radiologic features of acute epiglottis (A) compared with those of a normal airway (B).

Chapter 4
RESPIRATORY FAILURE

I.   OVERVIEW

A.   Definition
Any clinical condition marked by inadequate CO_2 elimination and/or inadequate oxygenation of blood.

B.   Etiologic Classification
Respiratory failure is divided into the two broad categories of lung failure and respiratory pump (or bellows) failure (Table 4-1).
1. Lung failure may develop from diseases affecting the airways, alveoli, alveolar capillary membranes, or pulmonary circulation and leads to hypoxemia and hypercapnia (Table 4-2 and 4-3).
2. Respiratory pump failure may arise from any disease along the pathway from the brain stem respiratory center to the upper spinal cord, phrenic nerves, and chest wall musculature and leads primarily to hypercapnia (Table 4-3).

TABLE 4-1. Respiratory Failure in Children: Common Causes

Lung Failure	Pump Failure
• Asthma	• Drug Overdose (*Chap. 11*)
• Bronchiolitis	• CNS Disease (*Chap. 9*)
• Bronchopulmonary dysplasia	
• Adult Respiratory Distress Syndrome	
• Upper airway obstruction (*Chap. 2, 3*)	

TABLE 4-2. Causes and Treatment of Hypoxemia

Physiologic Classification	Clinical Entities	Treatment
Low inspired O_2 concentration	• Disconnection from O_2 • High altitude	• Secure supplemental O_2 source
Hypoventilation	• Narcotic overdose • Sleep apnea • Brainstem injury	• Naloxone • Assisted ventilation
Low ventilation (V)/perfusion(Q) ratio	• Atelectasis • Pneumonia, Bronchiolitis • ARDS	• Chest physiotherapy • ↑ Lung volume with end expiratory pressure (PEEP)
Shunt ($^V/_Q = 0$)	• Cyanotic congenital heart disease • Severe atelectasis, ARDS	• Hyperventilation/Respiratory alkalosis • Prevent agitation • Surgical correction of cyanotic heart disease • Bronchoscopy to remove airway plug • PEEP • Extracorporeal membrane oxygenation
Low O_2 delivery to tissues	• Shock, anemia + Mild lung disease	• Blood transfusion • Inotropes • Supplemental O_2 and PEEP

TABLE 4-3. Causes and Treatment of Hypercarbia

Physiologic Classification	Clinical Entity	Treatment
↓ CO_2 elimination		
↑ V_D/V_T ratio (i.e., ↑ dead space, ↑ ventilation)	• Pulmonary embolism • Asthma, Bronchiolitis • Shock • Appartus attached to the airway - low fresh gas flow	• ↑ Pulmonary blood flow (↑ intravascular volume, inotropes, remove obstruction) • Bronchodilators • Assisted ventilation
↓ Minute ventilation	• CNS depression • Cervical cord injury • Myasthenia gravis • *Guillain-Barre* syndrome • Diaphragm fatigue	• Assisted ventilation • Anticholinesterase
↑ CO_2 production		
↑ Metabolic rate	• Hyperthermia • Sepsis • Hypertonic Dextrose	• ↑ Ventilation • Cooling, antipyretics • Dantrolene for malignant hyperthermia

C. Evaluation

1. Physical examination is the most important tool in the diagnosis of acute respiratory failure. Most patients have the typical picture of respiratory distress (Table 4-4). However, a small group of patients with pump failure may exhibit only hypoventilation and few signs of distress.

2. Pulse oximetry provides continuous information regarding a patient's oxygen saturation. An oxygen saturation $<90\%$ corresponds to a $PO_2 < 60$ mmHg. It implies that:

   (a) supplemental O_2 and possibly assisted ventilation is needed,

   (b) causes of respiratory failure should be sought, and

   (c) the patient must be monitored closely for further decompensation.

3. Laboratory tests include the arterial blood gas (Tables 4-4 and 4-5) and chest x-ray which may only show minor abnormalities and must be interpreted in the context of the physical exam. Example: The asthmatic child with PCO_2 of 40 mmHg and a clear chest x-ray may exhibit severe respiratory distress and impending respiratory failure.

TABLE 4-4. **Physical Exam and Arterial Blood Gas in Acute Respiratory Failure**

Signs & Symptoms	Blood Gas
• Tachypnea	• $PO_2 < 60$ mmHg (FIO_2 0.6)
• Chest Wall Retractions	• $PCO_2 > 45$ mmHg
• Diminished Breath Sounds	• pH < 7.3
• Cyanosis	
• Lethargy	

TABLE 4-5. Normal arterial blood gases in children (mean ± 2SD)

	Newborn (age 24 hrs.)	Infant (1-24 mos.)	Child (7-9 yrs.)	Adult
pH	7.37±.06	7.40±.06	7.39±.02	7.40±.03
$PaCO_2$	33 ± 6	34 ± 8	37 ± 3	39 ± 5
BE	-6.0 ± 3	-3.0 ± 3	-2.0 ± 2	0.0 ± 2
[HCO_3]	20 ± 3	20 ± 4	22 ± 2	25 ± 4

II. ASTHMA

A. Definition

Asthma is a chronic pulmonary disease characterized by recurrent episodes of acute lower airway constriction.

B. Pathophysiology

1. Neurogenic Factors
   a. Cholinergic (parasympathetic) stimulation leads to bronchial smooth muscle constriction and increased mucous production.
   b. Beta adrenergic (sympathetic) stimulation enhances smooth muscle relaxation and ciliary clearance and diminishes vascular permeability and bronchial edema.
2. Cellular mediators of inflammation (e.g., histamine, platelet activating factor) may aggravate bronchoconstriction, increase mucous secretion, and reduce mucociliary clearance.

C. Management

1. Initial Emergency Room (ER) Phase
   a. O_2 by nasal prongs or face mask.
   b. Nebulized bronchodilators (Table 4-6) are preferred over subcutaneous injection. However, if nebulization equipment is unavailable or the patient cannot cooperate with nebulization treatment, then terbutaline 0.01 mg/kg SC q 20 min x 3 may be given.
   c. Monitor heart rate and O_2 saturation.
   d. Advance therapy in ER if no improvement.

TABLE 4-6. Bronchodilator Agents for Nebulization (in 2.5 ml NS)[*]

Name	Concentration	Dose
Terbutaline (Brethine, Bricanyl)	1 mg/ml[**]	0.2 mg/kg (max 10 mg) q 30 min x 3
Metaproterenol (Alupent, Metaprel)	50 mg/ml	0.5 mg/kg (max 15 mg) q 30 min x 3
Albuterol (Ventolin, Proventil)	5 mg/ml	1st dose: 0.15 mg/kg (max 2 mg), then 0.05 mg/kg (max 2 mg) q 20 min
Atropine	1 mg/ml	0.01 mg/kg (min 0.1 mg, max 0.5 mg)

[*] Nebulizers driven with 5 - 10 L/min O_2
[**] Approved by FDA for parenteral use, but also effective as aerosol. Do not dilute further.

2. Advanced ER Phase
   a. Add steroids and aminophylline (Table 4-7)
   b. Chest x-ray: rule out pneumothorax and major atelectasis
   c. Admit to regular ward if improved.
   d. Admit to ICU if impending respiratory failure present.
   e. Intubate for imminent respiratory arrest (Table 4-13).

TABLE 4-7. Aminophylline and Steroid Protocol

IV Aminophylline
Loading Dose
- Theophylline level 0: 6-8 mg/kg
- Theophylline level >2 μg/ml: 1 mg/kg per μg desired rise in level

Infusion rate
- Infants: 0.65 mg/kg/hr
- Children: 0.9-1.1 mg/kg/hr

IV Steroids
- Hydrocortisone 4-6 mg/kg q 6h
- Methylprednisolone 1 mg/kg q 4-6h

---

3. ICU Phase - Major Problem: Hypercapnia (PCO_2 > 40 mmHg).
   a. Monitoring required for the asthmatic patient with hypercapnia includes ECG, respirations, pulse oximetry, and arterial line.
   b. Supplemental O_2 (30-60%) is applied by face mask. Two methods of nebulized bronchodilator administration may be employed:
      (1) A beta-2 sympathomimetic agent (metaproterenol, albuterol, terbutaline) is alternated with an

anticholinergic agent (atropine) every 15 min (Table 4-6); or

(2) a highly selective beta-2 agent (albuterol or terbutaline) is nebulized continuously.

c. Intravenous aminophylline and steroid administration is continued (Table 4-7).

d. If PCO_2 > 55 mmHg, then an isoproterenol infusion (0.1 μg/kg/min) is started and nebulized bronchodilators are stopped. If isoproterenol toxicity develops as manifested by heart rate > 200 or myocardial ischemia on ECG, then isoproterenol should be discontinued. In the absence of isoproterenol toxicity, the isoproterenol infusion rate is doubled every 15 min until the PCO_2 begins to fall.

e. Endotracheal intubation and mechanical ventilation are instituted under the following circumstances:

(1) Exhaustion of the patient,

(2) Isoproterenol toxicity or

(3) PCO_2 > 65 mmHg. (See also Table 4-13).

4. Major Problem: Hypoxia (PO_2 < 60 mmHg on FIO_2 0.6)

a. Supplemental O_2 administration, monitoring, and therapy with nebulized bronchodilators, aminophylline, and steroids proceed as described for the hypercapnic asthmatic patient.

b. The chest x-ray is reviewed carefully for pneumothorax and/or major atelectasis which may require chest tube drainage or bronchoscopy respectively.

c. If hypoxemia persists, add CPAP 5 - 10 cm H_2O by face mask. Endotracheal intubation and mechanical ventilation are employed, if FIO_2 .6 and CPAP 5 - 10 cm H_2O do not relieve hypoxemia (see also Table 4-13).

III. BRONCHOPULMONARY DYSPLASIA (BPD)

A. Definition
BPD is a chronic lung disease found in ex-premature infants who have suffered an acute lung disease in the neonatal period (usually hyaline membrane disease) requiring mechanical ventilation and supplemental oxygen.

B. Pathophysiology (Table 4-8)
1. Overview.
BPD involves damage to airways and alveolar-capillary units which may result in hypoxia, hypercapnia, increased airway resistance, and cor pulmonale.

TABLE 4-8. Pathophysiologic Mechanisms in BPD

O_2 Toxicity, Mechanical Ventilation, Recurrent Infection

Alveolar-capillary Damage:
- Alveolar coalescence
- Alveolar collapse
- Interstitial and alveolar edema

$\Downarrow$

Hypoxia and Hypercapnia

Airway Damage:
- Malacia
- Granulation tissue
- Smooth muscle hypertrophy

$\Downarrow$

Increased airway resistance
Increased work of breathing

$\Downarrow$

Cor pulmonale, Growth failure

---

2. Acute respiratory failure
   Infection, fluid overload, bronchospasm, mucous plugging, or tracheo-bronchial collapse may add acute respiratory failure to the existing chronic respiratory condition.

C. Management (Table 4-10)

1. Diagnosis of acute respiratory failure in the BPD patient depends on recognition of the usual signs and symptoms of respiratory distress. Parental history is very helpful in determining if the patient's condition is different from the usual baseline state. The arterial blood gas (Table 4-9) reflects acute and chronic respiratory failure with a partially compensated respiratory acidosis.
2. The status of the patient's airway determines the order of steps used in the management of acute respiratory decompensation in BPD (Table 4-8). Many patients with severe BPD will present with a tracheostomy which allows ready access to the airway for suctioning and institution of controlled ventilation. Patients without a tracheostomy may receive bronchodilator and diuretic therapy before proceeding to emergency intubation unless they exhibit evidence of impending respiratory arrest.

TABLE 4-9.   The Blood Gas in BPD: Acute and Chronic Respiratory Failure

---

- $PO_2 < 60$ mmHg ON FIO_2 60%
- PCO_2 20 mmHg OVER BASELINE
- pH < 7.30
- $HCO_3^- > 24$ mEq/L

TABLE 4-10.   Management Algorithm for BPD Patients with Acute Respiratory Failure

Without Tracheostomy	With Tracheostomy
• O$_2$	• O$_2$
• Nebulized Bronchodilators (Table 4-6)	• Suction Tracheostomy
• Methylprednisolone 2 mg/kg	• Nebulized Bronchodilators
• Consider furosemide 1 mg/kg	• Methylprednisolone 2 mg/kg
• Intubation & Ventilation (Table 4-13)	• Controlled ventilation via tracheostomy
• Cultures and Antibiotics	• Add sedation and paralysis
	• Consider furosemide 1 mg/kg
	• Cultures and Antibiotics

IV. BRONCHIOLITIS

A.   Definition

Bronchiolitis is an acute lower airway disease characterized by rhinorrhea, cough, low grade fever, wheezing, and tachypnea. The most common etiologic agent is the respiratory syncytial virus (RSV). Infants are most commonly affected and certain patient groups have a significantly increased mortality (Table 4-11).

TABLE 4-11.   RSV Bronchiolitis High Risk Patients

- Congenital Heart Disease
- BPD
- Prematurity
- Immunodeficiency

B. **Pathophysiology**

1. Lower airway obstruction secondary to mucosal inflammation and mucous plugging is the hallmark of bronchiolitis. This leads to hyperinflation and increased work of breathing.

2. Intrapulmonary shunting arises when there is bronchiolar obstruction and decreased ventilation to lung units which results in hypoxemia. Although patients also have increased deadspace ventilation, they are able to maintain normocapnia by breathing faster.

3. Fatigue occurs when the infant has been forced to increase work of breathing for prolonged periods. Fatigue is heralded by rising PCO_2 and worsening hypoxia.

4. Central apnea with complete absence of respiratory effort may develop suddenly and after only minor symptoms in young infants.

C. **Management**

1. Close observation and monitoring are recommended for infants with respiratory distress and infants in the high risk categories even if their distress is relatively mild.

2. Because of the high incidence of nosocomial spread of RSV bronchiolitis, infected patients should be cohorted and hospital personnel should observe strict handwashing before and after touching the patient.

3. Supplemental O_2.

4. Maintenance IV fluids after correcting dehydration.

5. Ribavirin administration is controversial. Ribavirin is an antiviral agent which is administered through a small particle aerosol generator. Virus shedding diminishes and subjective assessments of respiratory distress improve more rapidly in ribavirin treated patients. However, objective measures of outcome such as mortality, length of hospital stay, and need

for ICU care have not been shown to improve following ribavirin therapy. Ribavirin produces a small, physiologically insignificant improvement in arterial blood gases.

6. Steroids and bronchodilators may be tried in patients with a prior history of reactive airway disease.

V. ADULT RESPIRATORY DISTRESS SYNDROME (ARDS)

A. Definition

The Adult Respiratory Distress Syndrome (ARDS) is a syndrome of parenchymal lung injury characterized by hypoxia, diffuse pulmonary infiltrates, and decreased pulmonary compliance. Various triggering events may lead to the development of ARDS. The most common precipitating factors in children are given in Table 4-12.

TABLE 4-12. Common Pediatric Causes of ARDS

- Shock
- Sepsis, Pneumonia
- Near Drowning
- Aspiration

B. Pathophysiology

ARDS represents the final common pathway following a variety of pulmonary or extra-pulmonary insults.

The fundamental pathophysiologic abnormality appears to be disruption of the alveolar capillary membrane or an increase in permeability of the membrane. Activated granulocytes may release lysosomal proteases and oxygen free radicals which disrupt the alveolar-capillary membrane. Activated macrophages may discharge cytokines such as tumor necrosis factor (TNF) and interleukin-1 (IL-1), which, in turn, stimulate the release of prostaglandins that damage pulmonary vascular endothelium.

C. Management

1. Supplemental O_2 by mask (Table 2-2).
2. Fluid resuscitation to restore normovolemia (if necessary).
3. Broad spectrum antibiotics after blood culture.
4. Intubation criteria: Inability to maintain PO_2 > 60 mmHg on FIO_2 0.6 (see Table 4-13).
5. Following intubation apply continuous positive airway pressure (CPAP) 5 - 30 cm H_2O to prevent alveolar collapse.
   a. CPAP > 14 cm H_2O may be associated with hypotension.
   b. Measure central venous pressure, pulmonary capillary wedge pressure, and cardiac output to titrate supplemental fluid and inotropic drug administration.
6. Bronchoalveolar lavage or open lung biopsy if infectious pneumonia suspected.
7. Start mechanical ventilation with positive end expiratory pressure (PEEP) if patient becomes hypercapnic or PO_2 < 60 mmHg on FIO_2 0.6 and maximal CPAP therapy.
8. Steroids are not recommended in ARDS.

TABLE 4-13. Emergency Intubation (Rapid Sequence Induction)

Breathing:	bronchospasm	spontaneous	hypoventilation	apneic
Hemodynamics:	stable	unstable	stable	unstable
Mental Status:	awake	lethargic	lethargic	flaccid/coma
1. Oxygen	100%	100%	100%	100%
2. Bag/Mask Ventilation	no	no	yes	yes
3. Cricoid pressure applied by an assistant to prevent regurgitation				
4. Drugs:	Check intravenous line for proper function!			
Anticholinergic	Atropine 0.01 mg/kg (min 0.15 mg, max 1 mg) IV			none
Sedative	Ketamine 1 mg/kg or Midazolam 0.2 mg/kg IV			none
Relaxant	Succinylcholine 1 mg/kg or Vecuronium 0.2 mg/kg IV			none
5. **Place** endotracheal tube, **confirm** position by auscultation, **release** cricoid pressure.				
6. **Secure** tube with tape and obtain chest x-ray.				

Chapter 5
SHOCK AND
FLUID RESUSCITATION

I. INTRODUCTION

A. Definition
Shock is a syndrome of **acute** homeostatic derangement, of **various etiologies,** involving multiple organ systems, which ultimately causes failure of cellular metabolism.

SHOCK IS NOT NECESSARILY
DECREASED INTRAVASCULAR VOLUME

B. Classification

    1.   Hypovolemic
        a.   Vomiting/Diarrhea
        b.   Hemorrhage
    2.   Cardiogenic
    3.   Neurogenic
    4.   Septic

II. PATHOPHYSIOLOGY

A. Cardiac Function
Three relationships explain hypotension in shock.

    1.   Blood pressure = cardiac output x systemic vascular resistance (SVR).
        A reduction in cardiac output which cannot be compensated for by an increase in SVR will result in a reduction in blood pressure.
    2.   Cardiac output = stroke volume x heart rate
        Marked reductions in heart rate or stroke volume result in reduced cardiac output.

3. Stroke volume is determined by preload (ventricular end diastolic volume), afterload (systemic vascular resistance), and myocardial contractility.

B. Baroreceptor Response

Shock is a complex syndrome, evidenced by decreased tissue perfusion (Table 5-1). An apparent decrease in circulating volume and a fall in the systemic blood pressure are sensed by the central baroreceptors in the heart, aorta and carotid arteries. Humoral and autonomic compensatory mechanisms act to increase cardiac output, blood pressure, and heart rate as blood volume falls. Peripheral vascular constriction ("auto-amputation") leads to preferential regional blood flow to the brain and heart.

TABLE 5-1. Signs and Symptoms of Shock

Vasoconstriction	Pallor
Cold extremities	Sweating
Poor peripheral pulses	Ileus
Altered consciousness	Oliguria

C. Mediator Response

In all hypoperfusion states, multiple mediators amplify the damage initiated by hypovolemia, hypoxia and ischemia. These mediators include: complement, lipopolysaccharides, interleukins, the coagulation cascade, tumor necrosis factor, granulocytes, eicosanoids, platelet activating factor, leukotrienes, endorphins, and free radicals. Cell death results from these insults and mediator activity.

D. Microcirculatory Derangements (Table 5-2)

As shock progresses, cellular acidosis produces systemic metabolic acidosis. Fluid leaks from the capillaries to the interstitium, further depleting circulating volume and worsening the shock state. Peripheral vasodilatation and pooling results in a reduction in ventricular filling volume (preload) and a subsequent decrease in cardiac output (Starling mechanism). Myocardial response to circulating catecholamines is blunted which lowers heart rate and contractility. This contributes to multiple organ failure and eventual death (irreversible shock).

III. HYPOVOLEMIC SHOCK

A. Definition

Hypovolemic shock from intravascular volume depletion (hemorrhage, trauma, diarrhea, vomiting, renal loss, deprivation), leads to cellular hypoperfusion, metabolic acidosis and cell death. This is the most common cause of shock in children. Blood pressure is an insensitive index of hypovolemia (Table 1-1, 5-3). Profound failure of homeostasis in shock syndromes ULTIMATELY results in hypotension.

TABLE 5-2. Microcirculatory Alterations in Shock

- **ALTERED ENDOTHELIUM**

Plugged capillaries	Abnormal smooth muscle regulation
Altered interstitium	Arterio-venous shunting
Damaged barrier function	Coagulation cascade

- **ALTERED STARLING MECHANISM**
- **BLOOD VISCOSITY CHANGES**

TABLE 5-3. Age and Average Blood Pressures

Prematures	systolic 40 - 60	
Full term	75/50	
1-6 months	80/50	Approximate ranges:
6-12 months	90/65	Mean pressure $\pm$ 20% =
12-24 months	95/65	95% confidence limits
2-6 years	100/60	
6-12 years	110/60	Values for females are
12-16 years	110/65	approximately 5% lower
16-18 years	120/65	
Adult	125/75	

B. **Severe Dehydration from Vomiting and Diarrhea**

1. Assessment of severity is based on the physical examination (Table 5-4) and on measured weight loss.
2. The fluid deficit can be calculated by multiplying the assessed percentage of dehydration (Table 5-4) by the child's weight. For example, a 20 kg child who is 10% dehydrated has lost 10% of his body weight or 2,000 ml of fluid (100 ml/kg).
3. Three types of dehydration are described based on the measured serum sodium:
    a. Isotonic (130-150 mEq/L)
    b. Hyponatremic (<130 mEq/L))
    c. Hypernatremic (>150 mEq/L)
4. In hypotonic dehydration all the manifestations listed in Table 5-4 appear at lesser degrees of deficit. In hypertonic dehydration the circulating volume is relatively preserved at the expense of cellular water, and less circulatory disturbance is seen for a given amount of fluid deficit.

5. Laboratory tests confirming dehydration include: urine specific gravity ($\geq$ 1.030), BUN (> 20 mg/dl), creatinine (> 1 mg/dl), and a BUN: creatinine ratio > 20:1.

TABLE 5-4. Clinical Estimation of Dehydration

Dehydration (% Body Weight)	Clinical Observation
5%	• ↑ HR (10-15% above baseline) • Dry mucous membranes • Concentration of the urine • Poor tear formation
10%	• Decreased skin turgor • Oliguria • Soft, sunken eyes • Sunken anterior fontanelle
15%	• ↓ blood pressure, tachycardia, tachypnea • Poor tissue perfusion and acidosis • Delayed capillary refill

---

C. Fluid Management

The fluid management of a dehydrated patient requires immediate restoration of an effective circulatory volume, replacement of old and ongoing losses and provision of normal maintenance fluid and electrolyte requirements.

D. Calculation of Maintenance Fluid Requirements

Administer:

1. 4 ml/kg/hr for the first 10 kg of body weight (100 ml/kg/day);
2. 2 ml/kg/hr for the second 10 kg of body weight (50/ml/kg/day);
3. 1 ml/kg/hr for each additional kg of body weight (20 ml/kg/day).
4. 2-4 mEq/100 ml sodium; 2-3 mEq/100 ml K^+

EXAMPLE

Calculate the maintenance fluid requirements for a 35 kg patient.

	Per hour	Per day
1st 10 kg of weight	4 x 10 = 40	100 x 10 = 1000
2nd 10 kg of weight	2 x 10 = 20	50 x 10 = 500
over 20 kg (15)	1 x (35-20) = 15	20 x 15 = 300
	Total: = 75 ml/hr x 24 hrs	= 1800 ml/day

E. Electrolyte Composition of Body Fluids

1. Extracellular Fluid

The extracellular fluid space is approximately 20% of the body's weight (40% in the newborn), and is divided 3:1 between the interstitial (15% of body weight) and intravascular (5% of body weight) space. The sodium composition of extracellular fluid is approximately 140 mEq/L.

2. Intracellular Fluid

Intracellular water makes up approximately 40% of the body's weight. There is minimal sodium and 150 mEq of potassium/L.

F. Sodium Replacement may be calculated by the formula:

$([Na^+]_{desired} - [Na^+]_{present})$ x kg weight x 0.6 = $[Na^+]_{needed}$ in mEq.

G. Fluid Management in Moderate and Severe (Isotonic or Hyponatremic) Dehydration

1. In the first minutes, the child is resuscitated with 10-20 ml/kg of Ringers lactate in order to expand the extra-cellular fluid volume and perfuse the vital organs. Ringers lactate is the most nearly physiologic solution available. Patients with severe liver disease may be unable to metabolize the lactate load. Although normal saline is a satisfactory fluid replacement, it has the potential for causing hyperchloremic-acidosis.

2. Urine output, peripheral perfusion, blood pressure and pulse rate should guide volume replacement. In severe shock (> 15% dehydration), extremely rapid intravascular volume replacement with as much as 40 ml/kg is required.

3. One half of the calculated loss is replaced along with maintenance fluid over the next 8 hours. $D_5.45$ NS is the preferred solution. Add 20 mEq/L of potassium once urine output is established. Ongoing losses are replaced concurrently ("piggybacked") with a solution that matches the fluid being lost, usually Ringers lactate.

4. The remainder of the calculated loss is replaced along with maintenance fluid over the next 16 hours. $D_5.45$ NS with 20 mEq/L of potassium is the preferred solution. Ongoing losses are replaced as discussed above.

5. If a poor therapeutic response is noted or there is evidence of cardiac or renal (hemolytic-uremic syndrome) disease, central venous or pulmonary artery pressure monitoring may be required to guide fluid management.

6. The initial resuscitation bolus of Ringers lactate is not routinely counted in the calculations to correct deficit and maintenance needs.

EXAMPLE
Calculate the fluid requirements for a 20 kg child who is 10% dehydrated (Serum sodium 132).

Deficit   20 kg x 10% (or 100 ml/kg) = 2000 ml
Maintenance   (10kg x 4ml/kg/hr)+(10kg x 2ml/kg/hr)=60 ml/hr

Time	Administered Fluid
0-30 minutes	20 ml/kg Ringers lactate.
30 min-8 hours	1/2 the deficit (1000 ml) / 8 hours=125 ml/hr + maintenance fluids (60 ml/hr) or 185 ml/hr of $D_5.NS$ + 20 mEq/L potassium.
9-24 hours	1/2 the deficit (1000 ml) / 16 hours=63 ml/hr + maintenance fluids (60 ml/hr) or 123 ml/hr of $D_5.NS$ + 20 mEq/L potassium.

7. In symptomatic (seizures) hyponatremia (usually $[Na^+]$ < 115-120 mEq/L), a 3% hypertonic solution (0.5 mEq Na^+/ml) can be used to rapidly increase serum sodium to 125 mEq/L. Usually 4 ml/kg of 3% NaCl is administered over 10 minutes.

H. Hypernatremic Dehydration

1. Hypernatremic dehydration is caused by excessive water loss (Diabetes Insipidus, nephropathy, diarrhea, adrenal insufficiency) or by salt poisoning (boiled skim milk). In the former there is weight lost, in the latter weight increases.

2. The degree of dehydration is difficult to assess, because circulating volume is relatively preserved at the expense of cellular water.

3. Free water deficit can be **ESTIMATED** by assuming 4 ml/kg water deficit for every mEq that the serum sodium exceeds 145 mEq/L.

4. Slow rehydration (48-72 hr) is the rule. Rapid rehydration often results in serious neurologic complications, including seizures.
5. If the serum sodium is > 175 mEq/L and the cause is salt poisoning consider peritoneal dialysis. If the cause is excessive water loss, deficit replacement therapy should decrease serum sodium by 15 mEq/L/day.
6. Resuscitation is often required in the first hour (hypotension, poor peripheral perfusion). 10-20 ml/kg of a balanced salt solution is used, either Ringers lactate or normal saline.

I. Hemorrhagic Shock

Indices of perfusion such as pulse rate, capillary refill, blood pressure (Table 5-3), urine output, mentation, respiratory rate and the presence of orthostatic hypotension are used to classify hemorrhagic shock (Table 5-5).

J. Blood Replacement Therapy

The replacement of blood for the child in hemorrhagic shock begins as soon as possible. Although all blood products (cells, platelets, fresh frozen plasma) are potentially contaminated with virus (hepatitis, HIV), this should not deter its life saving use.

1. Fresh Whole Blood
    Fresh (< 48 hr) whole blood contains red blood cells, platelets, and clotting factors. When available and crossmatched, it is the ideal replacement product. Unfortunately it is rarely available and stored ("banked") blood components must be used (packed red blood cells, etc.) instead. A full cross match takes about one hour to accomplish.

TABLE 5-5. Classification of Hemorrhagic Shock

	I	II	III	IV
Estimated blood volume deficit	10-15%	20-25%	30-35%	>40%
Pulse (bpm)	>100	>150	>150	>150
Resp	nl	increased	tachypneic	tachypneic/ apneic
Capillary refill (sec)	<5	5-10	10-15	>20
Blood pressure	nl	decreased pulse pressure	decreased	severely decreased
Mentation	nl	anxious	confused	unconscious
Orthostatic hypotension	+	++	+++	+++
Urine output	1-3 ml/kg	0.5-1 ml/kg	<0.5 ml/kg	none

2. Packed Red Blood Cells

   Packed red blood cells are red cell concentrates with a hematocrit between 50 and 70%. There are no platelets and very little Factor V and VIII in this solution. To maintain shelf life, packed cells are stored in solutions that bind calcium. Potassium levels may be high.

3. Type-Specific Blood

   In life-threatening shock situations, type-specific blood can be given without a full crossmatch. The incidence of major transfusion reactions when type specific, uncrossmatched blood is given is 1:1,000.

4. Type "O" Blood

   If type specific blood is unavailable, type "O" blood is given. Type "O" positive blood may be used in males and type "O" negative blood is used in females to avoid Rh sensitization.

5. Blood Filters

   Intravenous-filtering devices should be used when blood transfusions are given in order to remove platelet and fibrin aggregates. Blood filtering reduces microembolization to the lungs and the potential for lung injury (ARDS).

6. Warming Blood

   Blood from the blood bank is refrigerated and should be warmed prior to or during transfusion. Cold blood is associated with a higher incidence of myocardial arrhythmias.

7. Massive Transfusions

   Packed red blood cells do not contain Factor V, VIII and platelets. Patients receiving massive blood transfusions (> 100 ml/kg, or, 1.5 blood volumes) develop dilutional thrombocytopenia and coagulopathies. Platelet transfusions are often necessary to treat this because they contain the depleted clotting factors as well as platelets.

8. Blood component replacement (Table 5-6)

   a. Red blood cells

Estimated blood volume (EBV) is calculated by equation 1.
1) EBV = Weight in kg x Blood Volume in ml (Table 5-6)

The volume of red blood cells for transfusion is calculated by equation 2.

$$2)\ \text{Volume of cells (ml)} = \frac{(EBV) \times (Hct_{desired} - Hct_{present})}{\text{Hematocrit (Hct) of Packed RBCs}}$$

TABLE 5-6. Intravascular Blood Volume

Age	Blood Volume
Premature	100 ml/kg
Term infant	90 ml/kg
Child	80 ml/kg
Adult	60-70 ml/kg

    b.   Platelet Transfusion
       (1) Give 4 units/M^2.
       (2) One unit of platelets per M^2 raises platelet count 10,000/mm^3 in absence of platelet destruction or antiplatelet antibodies.
       (3) Hemorrhagic complications are rare when platelet counts $> 20,000/mm^3$.

$$\text{Platelet increment/mm}^3 = \frac{30,000 \times (\text{number of units})}{\text{EBV (L)}}$$

    c.   Fresh Frozen Plasma (FFP)
       There are very few indications for this blood product. Coagulopathies following massive transfusions are usually caused by dilutional thrombocytopenia. FFP may be useful when treating disseminated intravascular coagulopathy (DIC).

9.   Calcium
    Packed red blood cells and platelets contain calcium binding agents. In massive transfusions hypocalcemia may produce hypotension. Calcium chloride 10 mg/kg, or calcium gluconate (30 mg/kg) is used in symptomatic patients or following transfusion of > 100 ml/kg of blood.

K. **Specific Therapy for Hemorrhagic Shock**

1. Class I

    Replace the volume loss with a balanced salt solution (Ringer's lactate or normal saline). Administer 10-20 ml/kg as a bolus, replacing 3 ml of crystalloid for every 1 ml of circulating blood volume lost. The rationale for the "3 for 1" rule is that only 1/3 of the crystalloid infused remains in the intravascular space.

2. Class II

    Class II hemorrhage is treated in the same way as Class I hemorrhage, except that blood is frequently required as well. Ongoing blood losses are replaced ml for ml with blood.

3. Class III, IV

    A Class III or IV hemorrhage requires blood as well as Ringer's lactate. Whole blood is preferred if it is available. If properly crossmatched blood cannot be given, type-specific or low titer "0" Rh⁻ blood is recommended. A pneumatic garment (MAST) may be necessary to raise blood pressure acutely (see section VII).

IV. CARDIOGENIC SHOCK

A. **Definition**

Cardiogenic shock is acute hypoperfusion and acidosis caused by heart failure. Causes include: congenital heart disease, trauma, infection, cardiomyopathies, Kawasaki's disease, and drug intoxications. The recognition of cardiogenic shock requires careful examination of the heart, ECG, chest x-ray and echocardiogram.

B. **Neonatal Pathophysiology**

Hypoplastic left heart syndromes (HLHS) (interrupted aortic arch, congenital aortic stenosis, etc) are common causes of cardiogenic shock in the newborn. The availability of palliative and corrective surgery make recognition of these syndromes imperative. Neonates with HLHS may survive the first weeks of life because the majority of aortic blood flow is supplied via the patent ductus arteriosus (PDA). Cardiogenic shock occurs when the ductus arteriosus closes. Because of this, any neonate in shock should immediately receive therapy to maintain ductus dependent flow (prostaglandin E_1 infusion, Table 5-7).

TABLE 5-7. Management of Hypoplastic L.H.S.

Cautious fluid administration, 5 - 10 ml/kg RL
Prostaglandin E_1 0.05 - 0.1 μg/kg/min
Mechanical ventilation
Bicarbonate for severe metabolic acidosis
Rule out sepsis

C. Management

1. Vasopressors (Table 5-8)
   The goal is to provide increased inotropy without excessively ↑ myocardial oxygen consumption.
   a. Dopamine 5-20 μg/kg/min
   b. Dobutamine 5-20 μg/kg/min
   c. Epinephrine 0.05-1 μg/kg/min

2. Fluids
   In the absence of jugular venous distension, pulmonary edema and hepatomegaly, Ringer's lactate in 5-10 ml/kg aliquots is given while monitoring perfusion. Fluid administration is stopped if no improvement in perfusion is noted **or** congestive symptoms develop (hepatomegaly, pulmonary edema, etc).

TABLE 5-8. Catecholamines Used in the Treatment of Shock

Drug	Mechanism				Dose μg/kg/min	Comments
	Alpha	Beta$_1$	Beta$_2$			
Epinephrine	+++	+++	+++		0.05–1.0	1. Positive inotrope and chronotrope. 2. Intense alpha effect at high dose, will ↓ peripheral tissue and organ (kidney and splanchnic) blood flow. 3. ↑↑ cardiac O$_2$ consumption.
Dopamine	At high dose	++	±		Low: 2–5 Mod: 5–15 High: ≥ 20	1. Low dose (dopaminergic): ↑ renal and splanchnic blood flow, minimal cardiac effect; often used in combination with dobutamine or epinephrine. 2. Moderate dose: ↑ chronotropy, inotropy, and cardiac output. 3. High dose: Intense alpha effect, will ↓ peripheral tissue and organ (kidney and splanchnic) blood flow.

Drug	Mechanism				Dose µg/kg/min	Comments
	Alpha	Beta₁	Beta₂			
Dobutamine	-	++	±		1-15	1. Positive inotrope, min chronotrope; ("weak isoproterenol"). 2. Administered in combination with dopamine.
Isoproternol	-	+++	+++		0.05-0.2	1. Positive inotrope and chronotrope. 2. Pure beta agonist, peripheral vaso- and bronchodilation. 3. ↑ cardiac O_2 consumption, which ↓ supply.
Norepi-nephrine	+++	+++	-		0.05-0.2	1. Positive inotrope. 2. Primarily alpha effect, will ↓ peripheral tissue and organ (kidney and splanchnic) blood flow.
Phenyleph-rine	+++	-	-		1-10	1. Pure alpha effect, will ↓ peripheral tissue and organ (kidney and splanchnic) blood flow.

D. Arrhythmias

An ECG is essential in all forms of shock to evaluate cardiac rate and rhythm. The presence of supraventricular tachyarrhythmias or ventricular tachycardia must be ruled out in all cases of hypoperfusion. Cardiac arrhythmias are discussed in *Chapter 7.*

V. NEUROGENIC SHOCK

A. Definition

Neurogenic shock is characterized by hypotension due to diminished or absent sympathetic activity and loss of vascular tone. The classic example is shock following transection of the cervical spinal cord.

B. Pathophysiology

Reduced peripheral vascular tone leads to pooling of blood in the extremities and inadequate venous return. Initially the patient has warm extremities, low diastolic pressure and a very wide pulse pressure. Ultimately perfusion pressure falls and acidosis develops.

C. Management
1. Trendelenburg position (head down, legs elevated)
2. Ringer's lactate or normal saline in 10-20 ml/kg aliquots.
3. Vasopressor drugs
    a. Phenylephrine (neosynephrine)
        (1) Action: Direct alpha adrenergic stimulation (vasoconstriction).
        (2) Dose: 1-10 μg/kg
        (3) Duration: 5-10 min
        (4) Continuous infusion: 1-10 μg/kg/min
    b. Ephedrine
        (1) Action: Indirect alpha and beta adrenergic stimulation.
        (2) Dose: 0.1-0.2 mg/kg

VI. SEPTIC SHOCK

A. Definition

Septic shock results from overwhelming bacteremia and/or septicemia (peritonitis, pneumonia etc.) (Table 5-9).

B. Pathophysiology

The clinical picture is similar to neurogenic shock except there is evidence of sepsis. The peripheral tissues are initially well perfused and warm. The pulse pressure is elevated and the diastolic pressure is low. Ultimately, perfusion fails and lactic acidosis develops. Unlike neurogenic shock, there will be accumulation of interstitial fluid and edema, especially in dependent tissues. Frequently there will be pulmonary and/or cerebral edema as a result of endothelial disruption.

TABLE 5-9. Septic Syndrome

- Clinical suspicion or evidence for infection
- Temperature instability (fever or hypothermia)
- Tachycardia/Tachypnea
- Impaired organ system function
  - peripheral hypoperfusion　　　　hypoxemia
  - altered level of consciousness　　acidosis
  - oliguria　　　　　　　　　　　　pulmonary edema

C. Management

1. Ringer's lactate is titrated in 10-20 ml/kg aliquots until the blood pressure <u>and</u> peripheral perfusion are restored to normal. This may require massive fluid administration (50-100 ml/kg).

2. Vasopressors (Table 5-8)
    a. Dopamine 5-20 μg/kg/min
    b. Dobutamine 5-20 μg/kg/min
    c. Epinephrine 0.05-1 μg/kg/min
3. Antibiotic therapy is dependent on the age of the patient (See *Chapter 12*). The neonate in shock requires acyclovir to treat for the potential of herpes simplex sepsis.

VII. SPECIAL TECHNIQUES IN SHOCK

A. Military Anti-Shock Trousers (MAST)

1. Indications/Contraindications
    Hypotension from shock of any etiology can be treated with the MAST. Indications include systolic BP < 70 mmHg in children > 2 years. The MAST provides a method of immediately shunting blood to vital organs, even before volume replacement can be given. It is useful for the control of intra-abdominal, pelvic and lower extremity bleeding. **Pulmonary edema** is the one absolute **contraindication** to the application of the MAST. Head trauma with coma is a <u>relative</u> contraindication.
2. Inflation
    The MAST is inflated until BP is adequate. Check valves in the suit will prevent over inflation.
3. Intravenous Fluid Replacement
    After application of trousers, large bore intravenous catheters are inserted above the trousers and Ringer's lactate and blood are given as needed.
4. Deflation/Removal
    The trousers are deflated in a gradual process starting with the abdominal segment. Deflation is stopped when blood pressure drops 5 mmHg. Intravenous fluid replacement is then increased. After the abdominal segment has been deflated, the

legs are each deflated in a similar fashion. If the patient requires transfer to another facility, the MAST is left on for transport.

B. Vascular Access (see also *Chapter 6*)

Vascular access must be obtained immediately. When IV access cannot be obtained within 1-2 minutes in children ≤ 5 years of age, use the INTRAOSSEOUS route of fluid (and drug) administration. In this technique, a Luer locked bone marrow needle is placed in the proximal tibial shaft (Figure 5-1). The intramedullary space is directly contiguous with the intravenous compartment, so that fluid and drugs readily pass to the central circulation following intraosseous administration.

C. Colloid Therapy

Large volumes of crystalloid can contribute to interstitial and pulmonary edema. Attempts have been made to decrease interstitial and pulmonary edema by supplementing Ringer's lactate with colloid infusions (albumin, fresh frozen plasma, and hydroxyethyl starch solutions). Although they have been shown to maintain intravascular volume longer than crystalloid infusions, there is little evidence that these increase patient survival. There is some evidence that hyperosmolar solutions containing RL and colloid may be the volume replacement of choice in hemorrhagic shock.

VIII. MONITORING

The treatment of shock requires adequate monitoring. Although pulse and blood pressure changes identify shock, other monitoring is essential. The most important monitors are those that indicate the quality of perfusion (Table 5-10).

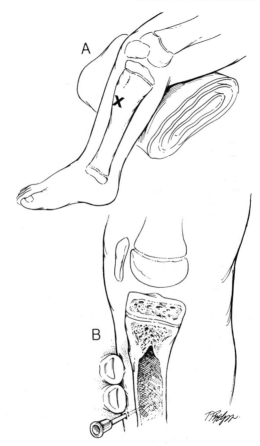

Figure 5-1. Intraosseous needle placement. Insert needle at the level of the tibial tubercle on the medial portion of the tibia. The needle is aimed caudally and laterally.

TABLE 5-10. Monitoring

•Pulse	•Respiratory Status
•Blood Pressure	•Urine - Foley
•Capillary Refill	•Blood Gases
•Toe temperature	•Central Venous Pressure
•Acid-Base balance	

A.   Toe temperature

The temperature of the great toe should be within 2 degrees (C) of the rectal temperature. The worse the state of perfusion the colder the toe and extremities become. The level of temperature demarcation (toe, foot, calf) can be used to guide the adequacy of resuscitation.

B.   Central Venous Pressure (CVP)

A central venous pressure catheter (or a pulmonary artery catheter) is placed when there is an inadequate response to the initial fluid challenges. The CVP reflects right ventricular compliance rather than volume. A poorly compliant ventricle may be volume depleted ("empty") and yet have a high filling pressure. Although right sided filling pressures usually reflect left heart function, there are certain conditions (pulmonary disease, mitral stenosis or positive pressure ventilation) when this is not true. When this occurs a pulmonary artery catheter to measure pulmonary artery occlusion pressure (PAOP) is needed.

Differential Diagnosis

1.   Elevated CVP (> 10 mmHg) or PAOP (> 12 mmHg)

   a.   tension pneumothorax

  b. pericardial tamponade
  c. cardiac failure (cardiogenic shock, myocardial insufficiency, myocarditis)
 2. Decreased CVP ($\leq$ 10 mmHg or PCWP ($\leq$ 12 mmHg) **and** poor perfusion
  Administer more crystalloid in 10 ml/kg aliquots. If the CVP does not increase by 3 mmHg after the infusion, give more crystalloid until either perfusion improves or the CVP rises by 3 mmHg.

IX. LABORATORY TESTS (Table 5-11)

Laboratory tests should be obtained in every patient in shock.

TABLE 5-11. Laboratory Tests

•Blood Sugar	•WBC & Differential
•Blood Gases	•Type and Cross
•Hematocrit	•Blood Cultures
	•Electrolytes

X. COMPLICATIONS

A. Continued Hemorrhage

When hemorrhage continues or is hidden, and fluid therapy produces a poor response, consider **immediate** surgical intervention.

B. Fluid Overload

Adequate volume replacement is absolutely essential to ensure survival and minimize damage. Capillary cellular damage accompanies shock which leads to fluid leak and interstitial edema. This occurs at normal intravascular volumes and pressures and is not a disease although it is frequently referred to as "volume overload." Intravascular hypervolemia should be avoided. Replace fluid to maintain tissue perfusion, normal intravascular pressures, and urine output at sufficiently low central venous pressures whenever possible.

C. Adult Respiratory Distress Syndrome (ARDS)

Pulmonary edema secondary to capillary leak occurs at normal cardiac filling pressures. Continued intravascular expansion may still be necessary to ensure adequate oxygen delivery even in the face of ARDS. When pulmonary edema develops, it is essential to know if left ventricular filling pressures are adequate. This requires pulmonary artery catheterization. The treatment of ARDS requires volume restriction and diuresis once hemodynamics and tissue perfusion have normalized. In more severe cases, when hypoxemia is not readily treatable by 60% inspired oxygen, airway intubation and mechanical ventilation with the addition of positive end expiratory pressure or CPAP are required (See *Chapters 2* and *4*).

D. Disseminated Intravascular Coagulopathy (DIC)

DIC is sometimes encountered, particularly in patients receiving > 100 ml/kg of blood. Preferred treatment modalities include fresh blood, platelets and fresh frozen plasma (FFP - 10 ml/kg).

E. "Failure to Respond"

When there is a failure to respond to administered therapy, consider:

1. ventilatory problems
2. unrecognized fluid loss
3. acute gastric distention
4. cardiac tamponade
5. myocardial contusion
6. diabetic acidosis
7. hypoadrenalism

Chapter 6
CARDIOPULMONARY RESUSCITATION

I. INTRODUCTION

Basic CPR for infants and children should follow the basic guidelines from the American Heart Association. The hierarchy of Airway, Breathing, and Circulation (ABC) describes the order of tasks during resuscitation of any critically ill infant or child. Table 6-1 compares techniques for infants and children.

II. ASSESSMENT

Basic CPR is instituted once apnea and pulselessness have been confirmed. The rescuer should look for chest excursions, listen for breathing, and feel for brachial or carotid pulses. If these findings are absent and the child is not immediately arousable, basic CPR is started.

III. ORGANIZATION

Effective resuscitation requires meticulous organization. This is simple when one or two rescuers are providing basic CPR, but becomes extremely complex during advanced CPR. The following roles should be clearly assigned and rehearsed during mock arrests in the hospital setting. The physician most experienced in resuscitation assumes overall command and coordinates the effort. A nurse supports the physician's efforts by obtaining the ordered medications and other materials (see *Chapter 21* for organization of equipment). The individual most skilled in airway management provides positive pressure ventilation with 100% O_2 via a mask or an endotracheal tube. A fourth person administers chest compressions. If this individual becomes physically exhausted, compression is taken over by relief personnel. Finally, a record keeper is needed to document all events, medications, and vital signs during the resuscitation. Excess personnel are very likely to hamper effective resuscitation.

TABLE 6-1. Basic CPR in Infants and Children

Infant	Older Child

Airway

Determine unresponsiveness

Call for help

Position patient supine.

Support head and neck.

Head-tilt/chin lift or Jaw thrust.

No blind finger sweeps.

Breathing

2 initial breaths

Then: **20** breaths/min	Then: **15** breaths/min

Circulation

Check **brachial** pulse	Check **carotid** pulse

Activate EMS System

Compression location: **1 finger breadth** below intermammary line on sternum	Compression location: **lower 1/3 of sternum**
Compression method: **Hands encircle chest or 2 fingers on sternum**	Compression method: **1 or 2 hands on sternum**
Compression depth: **0.5-1"**	Compression depth: **1-1.5"**
Compression rate: **100/min**	Compression rate: **80-100/min**

Compression:ventilation ratio = 5:1

Reassessment: Palpate pulse every 10 cycles

IV. AIRWAY MANAGEMENT FOR BASIC CPR

A. Positioning

Proper head, neck, and jaw positioning is designed to relieve airway obstruction usually caused by the tongue.

1. Head-tilt/neck-lift (Figure 6-1A)

    If there is no suspicion of neck trauma, the rescuer's hand is placed on the victim's forehead while applying firm backward pressure, to tip the head backward. Simultaneously the other hand is placed under the neck to lift and support it upward.

2. Chin-lift method (Figure 6-1B)

    The fingertips of one hand are placed under the mandible, bringing the chin forward which supports the jaw and tilts the head back.

3. Jaw-thrust (Figure 6-2)

    Provides additional forward movement of the jaw when the rescuer grabs the angles of the mandible and lifts with both hands, displacing the mandible and tilting the head backwards.

B. Mouth-to-Mouth Resuscitation

Rescue breathing is started once breathlessness has been confirmed.

1. Infants

    A tight seal is established by covering the infant's mouth and nose with the rescuer's mouth (Figure 6-3). The rescuer then breathes into the infant's mouth and nose twice while observing chest excursions.

2. Children

    If the rescuer's mouth does not cover the child's mouth and nose, a seal is accomplished by pinching the child's nose and covering the child's mouth with the rescuer's mouth (Figure 6-4). Rescue breathing is administered as above.

C. Foreign Body Obstruction

1. Evaluation

   Foreign body aspiration is suspected when the patient presents with choking, stridor, and cyanosis. There is often a history of the child playing with small objects prior to the choking spell. If the child is still breathing, no attempt is made to dislodge the foreign body. O_2 should be applied by face mask during transport. Conversely, if the patient is not breathing, the following emergency measures are instituted.

2. Management - Infants

   The infant is positioned over the arm of the rescuer with his head lower than the trunk. While providing support to the baby's head, four back blows are delivered rapidly with the heel of the hand between the infant's shoulder blades (Figure 6-5A). With persistent obstruction, the infant is turned over. His back is placed on the rescuer's thigh and four chest thrusts are delivered in rapid succession. Chest thrusts are given in the same manner chest compressions are performed (Figure 6-5B).

3. Management - Children

   Manual thrusts (Heimlich maneuver) are performed by standing behind the victim and wrapping one's hands around his waist (Figure 6-6). The rescuer grasps one fist with the other hand, places the thumb side of the fist against the victim's abdomen between the waist and the rib cage. In this position, the rescuer then presses his fist four times into the victim's abdomen with a quick inward and upward thrust. The unconscious victim is placed in the supine position. The rescuer faces the patient kneeling astride the patient's hips. With hands on top of each other, the heel of the bottom hand is thrust midway between umbilicus and xiphoid process in an inward and upward direction.

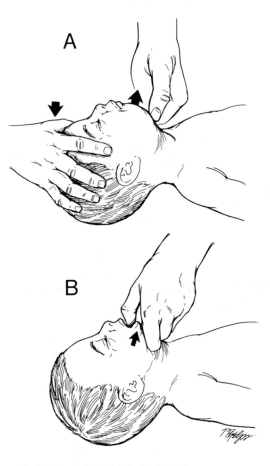

Figure 6-1. (A) Head tilt/Neck-lift; (B) Chinlift.
See Section IV for details.

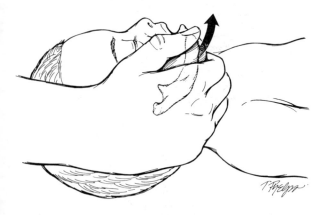

Figure 6-2. Jawthrust. The mouth is opened with the thumb and the mandible is elevated with the middle fingers.

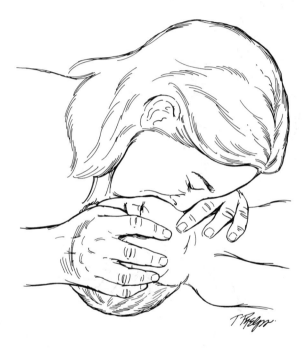

Figure 6-3. Mouth to mouth resuscitation in infants.
Rescuer's mouth is placed over victim's nose and mouth as the jaw is lifted.

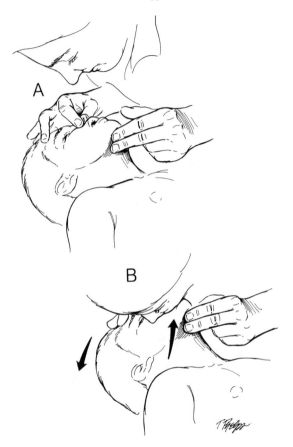

Figure 6-4. Mouth to mouth resuscitation in children.
(A) Nose is pinched. (B) Rescuer's mouth is placed over victim's mouth as the jaw is lifted.

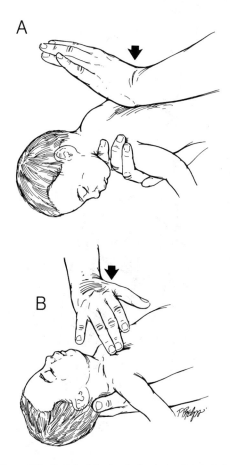

Figure 6-5. Relief of foreign body obstruction in infants.
(A) Backblows; (B) Chest thrusts.

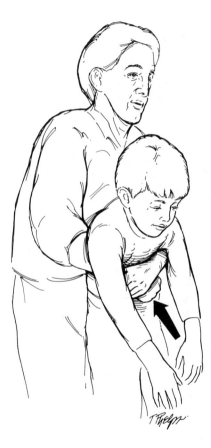

Figure 6-6. Relief of foreign body obstruction in children (Heimlich maneuver).

V. AIRWAY MANAGEMENT IN ADVANCED CPR

The critical step in escalating from basic to advanced life support occurs when 100% O_2 can be delivered by positive pressure ventilation. Positive pressure ventilation is achieved initially with a bag-valve-mask technique while cricoid pressure is applied to limit the risk of aspiration. The airway should be secured with endotracheal intubation as soon as possible to guarantee delivery of 100% O_2 and prevent aspiration (*Chapter 2*).

VI. CIRCULATION

A. Assessment

Absence of a pulse in the large arteries of an unconscious patient who is not breathing defines a cardiac arrest.

The brachial pulse is used to assess the presence of a pulse in an infant, the carotid pulse is used in the child.

B. Chest Compressions (Table 6-1)

1. Infant (Figure 6-7)
   a. Technique
      Two techniques may be used to compress the chest in infants. Two fingers are placed on the sternum one finger-breadth below the intermammary line. Alternatively, the hands encircle the chest, providing a firm surface to the back, and the thumbs are used to compress the chest at midsternum.
   b. Sternal compression depth: 0.5-1 inch.
   c. Compression rate: 100 times per minute.
   d. Compression:respiration ratio- 5:1.

2. Children (Figure 6-8)
   a. Technique
      The heel of the hand is placed two finger-breadths above the lower end of the sternum.
   b. Sternal compression depth: 1-1.5 inches.
   c. Compression rate - 80 times per minute.
   d. Compression:respiration ratio - 5:1.

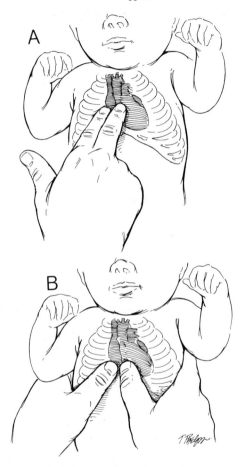

Figure 6-7. Chest Compressions in the infant.
(A) Two finger method; (B) Encircling method.

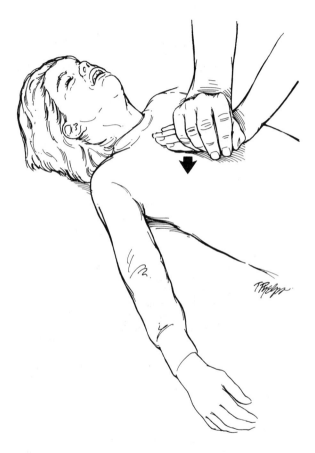

Figure 6-8. Chest compressions in the child.
See text on page 115 for description.

3. Physiology

The mechanism of blood flow during CPR is controversial. Initially, direct cardiac compression was felt to be responsible for blood flow during CPR. The intrathoracic pump mechanism has now been added as an additional explanation. In this mechanism blood flows because of the generalized increase in thoracic pressure when chest compressions are applied. Pressure is transmitted selectively into the arterial system because of effective valves in the jugular venous system. The resultant arterial to venous pressure gradient is responsible for blood flow.

C. Open-chest CPR

1. Indications

Although the vast majority of arrest situations call for closed chest CPR, there are certain specialized indications for thoracotomy to provide CPR (Table 6-2).

2. Technique

Resuscitative thoracotomy is most easily done in the operating room during surgical procedures involving the thorax. When this is done in the emergency room or intensive care setting, it can only be utilized by physicians familiar in this procedure. The heart should be placed between the thumb and second and third fingers and care should be taken not only to squeeze the heart adequately but also to allow refilling of the heart between direct compressions.

3. Physiology

Open-chest CPR is superior to closed-chest CPR in generating vital organ blood flow.

4. Risks

The risks include all of those associated with opening the chest (i.e., infection, ventricular rupture, residual pneumothorax, hemothorax).

TABLE 6-2. Indications for Open-Chest CPR following Cardiac Arrest

•Internal defibrillation, if external defibrillation is unsuccessful	•Chest or spine deformities (e.g., severe scoliosis) precluding effective closed chest CPR
•Stab wounds of the myocardium	•Left atrial myxoma or other intracardiac obstruction
•Massive air embolism	•Intrathoracic hemorrhage
•Ventricular or aortic aneurysms	•Cardiac arrest during an intrathoracic procedure
•Massive pulmonary embolism	

D. **Vascular Access Sites**

Advanced circulatory management requires vascular access (Table 6-3).

1. Children < 5 years old

A brief attempt is made to start an I.V. in the dorsum of the hands or feet or any other readily visible vein (Figure 6-9). If no access is achieved after 90 sec, an intraosseous needle is placed in the medial portion of the tibia at the level of the tibial tubercle (Figure 6-10). Longterm access is then achieved with either saphenous vein cutdown or a central vein line (e.g., femoral, external or internal jugular, or subclavian vein) (Figures 6-11, 6-12, 6-13, 6-14).

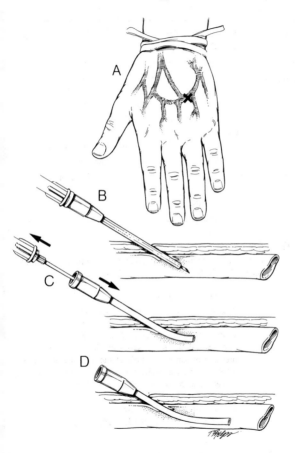

Figure 6-9. Peripheral venous access.
(A) Dorsum of the hand. (B,C,D) Sagittal view of the vein and catheter.

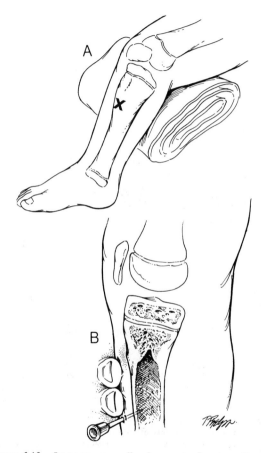

Figure 6-10. Intraosseous needle placement. Insert needle at the level of tibial tubercle on the medial portion of the tibia. The needle is aimed caudally and laterally.

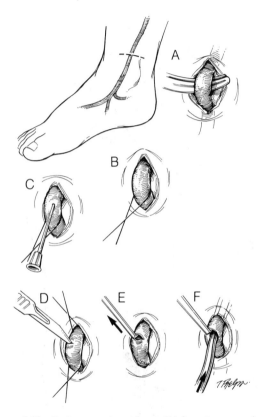

Figure 6-11. Saphenous vein cutdown. (A) 1 cm transverse incision medial to the medial malleolus. Blunt dissection with hemostat. (B) Control of vein with ligature. (C) Direct puncture with IV catheter or (D) proximal and distal control with ligature and incision with No. 11 scalpel blade. (E) Insertion of right angle vein guide. (F) Insertion of silastic catheter underneath vein guide.

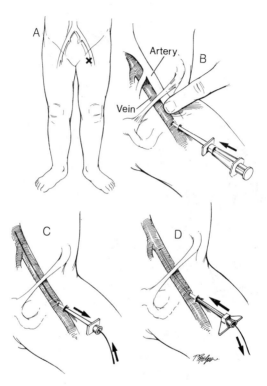

Figure 6-12. Femoral vein line placement (Seldinger technique). (A) Femoral vein midway between anterior superior iliac crest and symphysis pubis. (B) Insertion of needle into femoral vein just medial to femoral arterial pulse. (C) Insertion of guide wire through needle in the vein. Needle removed once guide wire in place. (D) Infusion catheter advanced over guide wire into vein. Guide wire removed after catheter in place.

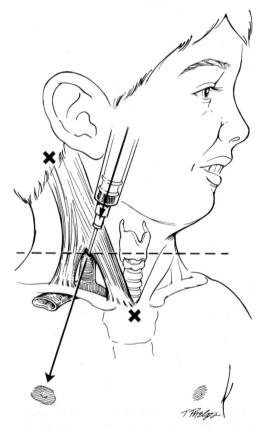

Figure 6-13. Internal jugular vein line placement. Head turned to the opposite side and needle puncture at the apex of the triangle formed by the heads of the sternocleidomastoid muscle (midway between the sternal notch and the mastoid process). Needle aimed at the ipsilateral nipple. Use Seldinger technique as in Figure 6-12.

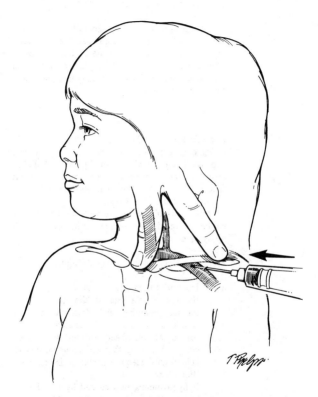

Figure 6-14. Subclavian vein line placement. Landmarks identified by placing operator's thumb in the sternal notch and index finger at the junction of the clavicle and 1st rib. Needle puncture 1 cm lateral and 1 cm inferior to clavicle-rib junction aiming for the sternal notch. Then use Seldinger technique (Figure 6-12) for line placement.

2. Children > 5 years old

    Peripheral venous access is generally easier in the
    older child and intraosseous needles are more
    difficult to place because bone cortex is thicker.
    Therefore, if peripheral I.V. placement fails, a
    saphenous vein cutdown or central line placement
    should be attempted.

3. Initial Fluid Administration

    Lactated Ringers solution or normal saline 10-20
    ml/kg over 2-5 min. A rapid 10 ml/kg volume
    expansion is justified in virtually every pediatric
    arrest scenario unless massive congestive heart
    failure (e.g., myocarditis or hypoplastic left heart
    syndrome) caused the arrest.
    A stopcock is placed in line with the I.V. tubing
    so that a titrated fluid volume can be administered
    by syringe.

4. Fluids for Hypovolemic Arrest (*Chapter 5*)

    a. Interstitial fluid loss
        If hypovolemia caused the arrest (e.g.,
        trauma, vomiting and diarrhea, sepsis),
        additional aliquots of lactated Ringers
        solution or normal saline 10 ml/kg are given
        every 2-5 min together with epinephrine (see
        below) until adequate perfusion is restored.
    b. Blood loss
        If hypovolemia was caused by blood loss,
        lactated Ringers solution should be changed
        promptly to type O Rh⁻ uncrossmatched
        whole blood or packed red cells. Type
        specific blood should be available from the
        blood bank in 15-20 min after receipt of a
        blood sample for type and cross match. A

spun hematocrit is checked initially and then every 30 minutes to monitor red cell administration (See *Chapter 5*).

c. Total fluid volume administration
There is no arbitrary maximum fluid volume in the face of hypovolemic arrest. Fluid and blood administration is titrated to restore an adequate blood pressure. Ongoing fluid losses must be subtracted from the administered volume to determine the net fluid volume. Pulses, breath sounds, liver size, peripheral edema, and skin color are constantly reassessed.

5. Dextrose Administration
The routine crystalloid fluid is isotonic and does not contain dextrose, because hyperglycemia may aggravate neuronal injury. However, glucose determination (Chemstrip) is checked to rule out hypoglycemia. If the Chemstrip <60 mg% D_{25}/W 4 ml/kg is given and D_5/1/4 normal saline is added at a maintenance rate, Chemstrips are then rechecked every 30 min.

6. Maintenance Fluids during CPR
Once intravascular volume has been restored, subsequent fluid administration should be reduced to 2/3 maintenance rates because of the likelihood of tissue edema. Because hypovolemia may recur, constant reassessment is necessary.

TABLE 6-3. Vascular Access Management During CPR

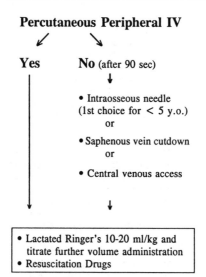

Percutaneous Peripheral IV

Yes   No (after 90 sec)

- Intraosseous needle
  (1st choice for < 5 y.o.)
  or
- Saphenous vein cutdown
  or
- Central venous access

- Lactated Ringer's 10-20 ml/kg and
  titrate further volume administration
- Resuscitation Drugs

VII. DRUGS

A. Route

1. Intravenous or intraosseous routes are the
    preferred routes for drug administration. All
    drugs which are effective intravenously are also
    effective intraosseously with virtually no delay in
    onset time.

2. Endotracheal administration of drugs
   The use of non-venous routes for administration of some drugs is possible via the endotracheal tube. **Epinephrine, lidocaine, naloxone,** and **atropine** can be administered through the endotracheal tube in the same doses as employed via the intravenous route. If intravenous or intraosseous access is delayed beyond 2-3 minutes, the above drugs should be given via endotracheal tube.

3. Intracardiac Administration
   The intracardiac route is hazardous (coronary artery laceration) during CPR and should be used only when no other routes are available.

B. Epinephrine

1. Physiology
   Epinephrine is an alpha and beta agonist. The alpha adrenergic effects are responsible for its beneficial impact during CPR. These cause a generalized vaso-constriction of peripheral vasculature resulting in an increase in coronary and cerebral blood flow (Table 6-4).

2. Indications
   a. Asystole
   b. sinus or junctional bradycardia
   c. fine ventricular fibrillation

3. Dosage
   a. Initial Dose- 10 μg/kg
      0.1 ml/kg of 1:10,000 solution
   b. If the initial dose is unsuccessful, double the dose on subsequent tries up to 100 μg/kg.

4. Supply
   a. 1:10,000 solution (100 μg/ml) premixed resuscitation syringe
   b. 1:1,000 solution (1 mg/ml) - ampules must be diluted 1:10 with normal saline

---

TABLE 6-4. Alpha and Beta Adrenergic Effects During CPR

Alpha-Adrenergic Effects
Advantages
- vasoconstricts peripheral vascular beds
- increases diastolic pressure → increases coronary blood flow
- constricts extracerebral carotid vessels → increases intracerebral blood flow

Beta-Adrenergic Effects
Advantages
- increases vigor of ventricular fibrillation
- positive inotrope and chronotrope
Disadvantages
- increases O_2 demand of tissues (i.e., heart and brain)
- increases arrhythmias following resuscitation

---

  5. Route of Administration
    Intravenous, endotracheal, intraosseous
  6. Effects
    a. Alpha, beta-1, beta-2 stimulation
    b. vasoconstriction
    c. positive inotropy, chronotropy
    d. increased intensity of ventricular fibrillation
    e. increased myocardial oxygen requirements

C. Sodium Bicarbonate (HCO_3^-)

  1. Physiology
    Bicarbonate is a buffer used to treat metabolic acidosis according to the reaction:
    $$HCO_3^- + H^+ \rightleftarrows H_2CO_3 \rightleftarrows H_2O + CO_2$$
    Effective treatment of metabolic acidosis requires
    a. effective pulmonary blood flow (i.e., effective chest compressions) so that the

metabolic product of the above reaction, namely CO_2, can be delivered from peripheral tissues to the lungs;

b.   effective ventilation so that accumulated CO_2 can be excreted by the lungs.

Unless these two requirements are fulfilled, bicarbonate administration will lead to tissue CO_2 accumulation and hence a combined respiratory and metabolic acidosis in the tissues including the myocardium, which may delay recovery of spontaneous cardiac activity.

2.   Indications

Because of the physiologic considerations outlined above, bicarbonate should be limited to cardiac arrest associated with:

a.   hyperkalemia,

b.   preexisting metabolic acidosis,

c.   After cardiac compressions, defibrillation, support of ventilation and anti-arrhythmics have been given (approximately 10 minutes into routine cardiac arrest sequence).

3.   Dosage: 1 mEq/kg or

Bicarbonate (mEq) = 0.3 x body weight (kg) x base deficit

4.   Route of administration

Intravenous, Intraosseous

5.   Effects

Increased pH

6.   Potential adverse effects of bicarbonate

a.   Hypernatremia

b.   Hyperosmolality

c.   Shift O_2 dissociation curve to left and hence reduced O_2 unloading in peripheral tissue.

d.   No proven positive effect in clinical situations.

e.   Did not offer benefit in defibrillating dogs compared to saline.

(Guerci, et al: Circulation 74:V75, 1986)

    f.   Deleterious in treating lactic acidosis
        (Graf, et al: Science 227:754, 1985)

    g.   CNS acidosis
        CO_2 formed by dissociation of bicarbonate rapidly enters neurons with slower egress of H^+ from cell.

D.　Atropine

1.　Pathophysiology
Because of the exaggerated effects of vagal stimulation in children, atropine is recommended in most pediatric arrest situations.

2.　Indications
Atropine is specifically indicated in sinus or junctional bradycardia, and in slow idioventricular rhythms.

3.　Dosage
    a.   0.01 mg/kg; minimum dose 0.15 mg (Paradoxical bradycardia may occur with smaller doses.)
    b.   maximum dose 1 mg

4.　Route of Administration
intravenous, intraosseous, subcutaneous, endotracheal, intramuscular

E.　Calcium Chloride

1.　Physiology
Calcium is essential for myocardial excitation-contraction coupling. Its major effect is to increase myocardial contractility and it may increase ventricular automaticity during asystole.

2.　Indications
Recent research suggests detrimental effects of calcium accumulation following ischemia and the possible benefit of calcium blockers to vital organs during resuscitation. Thus specific indications for calcium administration during CPR include:

    a.   Documented Hypocalcemia
- (1) Decrease in total body calcium (e.g., hypoparathyroidism, renal failure, pancreatitis)
- (2) Decreased ionized Ca^{++} (e.g., following massive blood transfusion)

    b.   Hyperkalemia

    c.   Hypermagnesemia

    d.   Calcium-Channel Blocker Overdose

3. Dose
   a. 10 mg/kg of calcium chloride
      0.1ml/kg of 10% solution
   b. 30 mg/kg of calcium gluconate

4. Route
   a. Calcium gluconate may be given via a peripheral vein or intraosseously.
   b. Calcium chloride should be given via a central vein.

5. Adverse effects
   May prevent reflow of blood into ischemic areas of the heart and brain.

F. Lidocaine

1. Indications
   Ventricular tachycardia

2. Dose
   a. 1 mg/kg
   b. If repeated doses are needed, an infusion of 20-50 μg/kg/min should be started.

3. Route
   Intravenous, intraosseous, endotracheal

G. Defibrillation

1. Physiology
   Ventricular fibrillation is characterized by random depolarization of myocardial cells. Defibrillation results in spontaneous depolarization of all

myocardial cells. A single pacemaker may then emerge to allow organized depolarization of the heart.

2. Indications
Ventricular fibrillation or ventricular tachycardia. The use of early defibrillation is critical in the cardiac arrest situation. Early attempts at defibrillation increase the likelihood of return of spontaneous electrical activity of the heart. The use of antiarrhythmics should never preclude defibrillation when the patient is hemodynamically unstable.

3. Dose: Ventricular fibrillation
   a. 2 J/kg (for ventricular fibrillation)
   b. If unsuccessful, check oxygenation, acid-base status, give epinephrine, double energy output and repeat defibrillation.

4. Dose: Ventricular tachycardia
Administer 0.5J/kg for ventricular tachycardia with hemodynamic instability and unresponsiveness to lidocaine and synchronized cardioversion. (See *Chapter 7.*)

5. Placement options
   a. One paddle on right upper chest quadrant; the other paddle to the left of the left nipple in anterior axillary line. OR
   b. One paddle anteriorly or over left precordium; the other posteriorly on the left upper back (behind the heart).

6. Paddle Size
   a. Infants - 4.5 cm
   b. Children - 8 cm
   c. Adults - 14 cm

VIII. ELECTROMECHANICAL DISSOCIATION

Electromechanical dissociation (EMD) is defined as organized electrocardiographic activity without evidence of myocardial contractions. The causes and therapy for EMD are given in Table 6-5.

TABLE 6-5. Causes and Treatment of EMD

Cause	Treatment
Cardiac (primary EMD): • Prolonged cardiac arrest • Massive infarction	Usually refractory to treatment • Epinephrine; other alpha-agonists • Calcium chloride • Atropine
Noncardiac (secondary EMD): • Hypovolemia • Pericardial tamponade • Tension pneumothorax • Pulmonary embolism	Usually successful. Treat underlying problem.

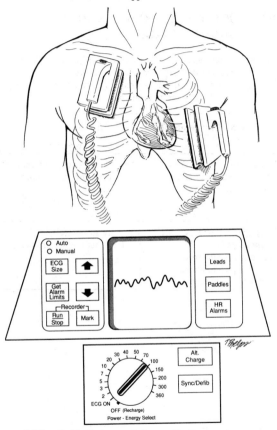

Figure 6-15.   Defibrillation technique. (1) Energy dose set at 2 joules/kg. (2) Apply gel to paddles and charge defibrillator. (3) Place one paddle on right upper chest and the second paddle between left nipple and left anterior axillary line. (4) Clear the bed. (5) Press discharge buttons on paddle.

Chapter 7
CARDIAC ARRHYTHMIAS

I. OVERVIEW
Cardiac arrhythmias are uncommon in children compared to adults, but may be just as life threatening. Their prompt recognition and treatment are essential.

II. PREDISPOSING FACTORS
Differential diagnoses to consider when evaluating the etiology of an arrhythmia are contained in Table 7-1.

III. EVALUATION

A. Hemodynamic Stability
Reestablishing hemodynamic stability is the primary goal of arrhythmia management. The origin of the arrhythmia may be of intellectual interest and of ultimate prognostic importance, but it should not detract the physician from treating a hypotensive patient.

B. Analysis of Atrial and Ventricular Impulses
The diagnosis of the arrhythmia requires analysis of both atrial and ventricular activity and the sequence of this activity. In very fast heart rates, atrial activity may be difficult to appreciate since p waves may not be visible in the ECG. Wide and bizarre QRS complexes suggest a ventricular origin in most cases. However, supraventricular origin with aberrant conduction may also produce wide QRS complexes. Rate dependent right bundle branch block is common in supraventricular arrhythmias.

IV. BRADYARRHYTHMIAS

A. Sinus Bradycardia (Figure 7-1A)
1. Characteristics
   Slow sinus rate (often as low as 30-60 beats per minute).

TABLE 7-1. Factors Predisposing to Arrhythmias

Congenital Heart Disease
- Atrial arrhythmias: Ebstein anomaly, atrial septal defects
- Atrial and ventricular arrhythmias: Anomalous left coronary artery (may also present with heart block)
- Supraventricular arrhythmias: L-transposition of the great arteries (may also present with heart block)

Isolated Conduction System Disorders
- Wolff-Parkinson-White syndrome
- Jervell-Lange-Nielsen syndrome (deafness and prolonged QT intervals)
- Romano-Ward Syndrome (prolonged QT interval without deafness)
- Maternal history of collagen vascular disease (systemic lupus erythematosus)

Associated with Systemic Illness
- Kawasaki disease (mucocutaneous lymph node syndrome)
- Friedreich's ataxia (atrial tachycardia or fibrillation)
- Muscular dystrophies (Duchenne, periodic paralysis)
- Glycogen storage diseases (Pompe disease)
- Collagen vascular diseases (rheumatic carditis, rheumatic arthritis, lupus, periarteritis nodosa, dermatomyositis)
- Endocrine disorders (hyperthyroidism, adrenal dysfunction)
- Metabolic and electrolyte disturbances (renal disease, beriberi)

Drug Toxicity
- Chemotherapeutic agents (adriamycin)
- Tricyclic antidepressants
- Cocaine
- Digitalis, beta blockers
- Asthma medications (sympathomimetics, aminophylline)

Other causes
- Blunt chest trauma (myocardial contusion)
- Increased intracranial pressure

---

2. Etiology
   a. Normal children.
   b. Vagal stimulation (e.g., during intubation in newborns).
   c. Hypoxia and hypotension
   d. Other causes include: drug toxicity (digitalis, beta-blockers, calcium channel blockers), hypothermia, increased intracranial pressure, and hyperkalemia.

3. Course
   Sinus bradycardia is of no consequence in the well trained athlete. Conversely, it may become the setting of an unstable nodal or ventricular escape rhythm. If underlying disorders such as hypoxia or hyperkalemia are not corrected, sinus bradycardia may degenerate into full cardiac arrest.

B. First Degree Atrio-ventricular (AV) Block (Figure 7-1B)

1. Characteristics
   First degree AV block is defined by **prolongation of the PR interval** beyond the limits for age and heart rate (infants > 0.14 sec; children > 0.16 sec; adolescents > 0.18 sec). The rhythm is regular, originates in the sinus node and has a normal QRS morphology.

2. Etiology
   Conduction through the AV node is delayed as manifested by the prolonged PR interval. First degree AV block may be seen in the following conditions:
   a. Healthy children
   b. Congenital Heart Disease
      (1) Atrial septal defect
      (2) Ebstein anomaly
   c. Acquired Heart Disease
      (1) Rheumatic fever
      (2) Cardiomyopathy

          d.   Drug toxicity
                (1)   Digitalis
                (2)   Beta blockers

3.   Course

The rhythm itself does not lead to hemodynamic compromise. However, it may be a sign of underlying heart disease. No specific therapy is required for first degree heart block. However the possibility of underlying heart disease should be evaluated and treated if necessary. First degree AV block should be ruled out before digitalis administration.

C.   Second Degree AV Block

Second degree AV block may be divided into Mobitz Type I, Mobitz Type II, or fixed ratio ("high degree") block. All types of second degree AV block have the following features in common: Some, but not all, atrial impulses fail to conduct to the ventricle and hence the atrial rate exceeds the ventricular rate.

1.   Mobitz Type I (Wenckebach Block)(Figure 7-1C)
        a.   Characteristics
             (1)   Progressive prolongation of the PR interval occurs over several beats until a QRS is dropped. This cycle repeats itself, although the number of beats in a cycle may not be constant.
             (2)   QRS configuration is normal.
        b.   Etiology
             (1)   Conduction disturbance at the level of the AV node.
             (2)   Same conditions as for first degree AV block.
        c.   Course

There are usually no hemodynamic disturbances associated with Wenckebach block alone. The course is similar to the one described for first degree AV block.

2. Mobitz Type II (Figure 7-1D)
   a. Characteristics
      (1) Sudden AV conduction failure with QRS dropped after normal p wave.
      (2) No preceding PR interval prolongation in normal, conducted beats.
      (3) QRS may be prolonged.
   b. Etiology
      Disease in the His-Purkinje system causes Mobitz Type II block.
   c. Course
      This is a more serious arrhythmia than first degree heart block or Wenckebach, because it may progress to complete heart block. Therapy must be individualized. Those patients with serious underlying heart disease and Mobitz Type II block might not tolerate progression to complete heart block and prophylactic pacemaker implantation should be considered.

3. Fixed Ratio AV Block (usually 2:1, may be 3:1 or 4:1) (Figure 7-1E)
   a. Characteristics
      (1) QRS follows only after every 2nd (3rd or 4th) p wave causing 2:1 (3:1 or 4:1) AV block.
      (2) Normal PR interval in conducted beats.
      (3) Normal or prolonged QRS.
   b. Etiology
      Either the AV node or the His bundle may be the site of injury to the conduction system. Intracardiac recordings are used to distinguish the site of conduction disturbance.
   c. Course

Progression to complete heart block may occur. Symptomatic patients (syncope, heart failure) require pacemaker placement.

D. Third Degree (Complete) AV Block (Figure 7-1F)

1. Characteristics
   a. No atrial impulses are conducted to the ventricle.
   b. Atrial rhythm and rate are normal for the patient's age.
   c. Ventricular rate is slowed markedly (40-55 beats/min).
   d. QRS may be of normal duration (escape rhythm arising in AV node) or QRS may be prolonged (escape rhythm arising in distal His bundle or ventricle).

2. Etiology
   a. Congenital complete AV block
      (1) Isolated abnormality
      (2) Associated with Transposition of the Great Arteries
      (3) Associated with maternal collagen vascular disease
   b. Open heart surgery (e.g., large ventricular septal defect closure)
   c. Cardiomyopathy

3. Course
   a. Newborns with congenital complete heart block may present with heart failure (hydrops fetalis). They suffer an increased risk of dying during the first year of life, especially if the ventricular rate is <55 beats/min and/or the QRS is widened.
   b. Complete heart block after open heart surgery may appear in the early postoperative period, but is usually transient (<2 weeks).

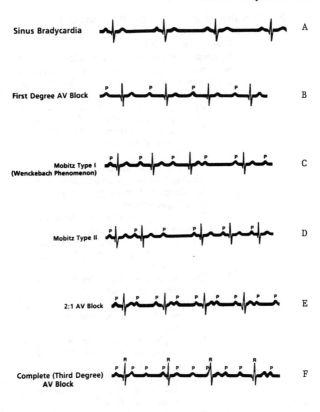

Figure 7-1. Bradyarrhythmias. (A) Sinus Bradycardia; (B) First Degree Atrioventricular (AV) Block; (C) Mobitz Type I (Wenckebach) 2nd Degree AV Block; (D) Mobitz Type II 2nd Degree AV Block; (E) 2:1 AV Block; (F) Third Degree (complete) AV Block.

E. Treatment Principles for Bradyarrhythmias

1. Treat the underlying cause

   Hypoxia, electrolyte abnormalities, drug intoxication, hypothermia, and increased intracranial pressure may precipitate or aggravate bradyarrhythmias.

   a. Ensure adequate oxygenation and ventilation. The majority of severe sinus bradycardias respond to improved oxygenation alone.

   b. Treat drug toxicity

      Withhold further administration of digitalis, beta-blockers, and calcium channel blockers. See *Chapter 11* on Drug Intoxication.

   c. Treat hyperkalemia.

      Signs of hyperkalemia include peaked T waves and QRS prolongation.

      (1) Calcium chloride 10 mg/kg or Calcium gluconate 30 mg/kg IV slowly

      (2) Bicarbonate 1 mEq/kg IV. Flush IV line carefully after calcium administration, because calcium and bicarbonate precipitate in the same solution.

      (3) D_{25}/W 1-2 ml/kg/hr and regular insulin 0.1 unit/kg/hr. Check serum glucose q 1h.

      (4) Kayexalate (sodium polystyrene resin) 1-2 gm/kg with 3-5 ml sorbitol/gm resin PO or PR q 6h.

   d. Treat hypothermia (See *Chapter 13*).

   e. Treat increased intracranial pressure (See *Chapter 15*).

2. Pharmacologic Measures

   Symptomatic patients with sinus bradycardia, second or third degree heart block require emergency measures to increase heart rate and cardiac output. Patients with normal QRS configuration usually respond to atropine or isoproterenol.

a. Atropine 0.01 mg/kg (min 0.15 mg, max 1 mg)
b. Isoproterenol infusion 0.1-1 μg/kg/min

3. Temporary atrial pacing
a. Indications
Sinus bradycardia or sick sinus syndrome (with normal AV node function) require pacing if treatment of the underlying cause or pharmacologic measures do not result in improvement.
b. Esophageal pacing
A standard transvenous pacing electrode is inserted into the esophagus until atrial capture can be achieved.

4. Temporary pacing of the right ventricle
a. Indications
The patient with 2nd or 3rd degree heart block who remains symptomatic despite pharmacologic measures requires temporary ventricular pacing until the underlying condition is corrected or a permanent pacemaker has been implanted. Typical pacemaker settings for temporary right ventricular pacing are shown in Figure 7-2. The following placement options exist:
b. Transvenous pacing (Figure 7-3)
A pacing electrode is inserted through an introducer in any central vein. If the pacing electrode is balloon-tipped, the balloon is inflated in the right atrium and deflated once the electrode has advanced into the ventricle. The electrode is connected to a grounded ECG, so that proper position in the apex of the right ventricle can be identified when ST segment elevation is

noted. Asynchronous pacing of the right ventricle is then instituted.

c. Pacing pulmonary artery catheter

Some pulmonary artery (Swan-Ganz) catheters have incorporated pacing electrodes to allow ventricular or AV sequential pacing. Generally, this technique is useful only in adolescent patients, because the ventricular electrode is likely to end up in the atrium in smaller patients after the tip of the catheter has been positioned in the proximal pulmonary artery.

d. Transcutaneous pacing (Figure 7-4)

Large cutaneous stimulating electrodes are placed on the anterior chest wall and on the back. Pacemaker output is gradually increased until ventricular capture is achieved. There is a risk of skin burn with cutaneous electrodes.

e. Transthoracic pacing (Figure 7-5)

A long spinal needle is inserted via a subxiphoid approach into right ventricle following puncture through the chest wall. The pacing electrode is then inserted through the needle until it is anchored in the apex and ventricular capture is achieved. This procedure should be employed only for pacing during full cardiac arrest.

f. Epicardial pacing

Following cardiac surgery, epicardial pacing wires are placed to permit either ventricular pacing or AV sequential pacing. AV sequential pacing is used, when the atrial contribution to cardiac output is needed. Immediate pacing is instituted for symptomatic or potentially hazardous bradycardia while eliminating the underlying cause if possible.

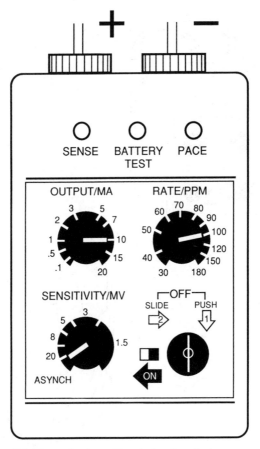

Figure 7-2. Pacemaker box with typical settings for temporary right ventricular pacing in an infant: Rate: 100/min, Sensitivity: Asynchronous, Output: 10 MA.

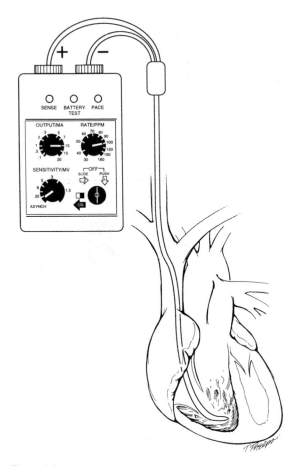

Figure 7-3. Transvenous pacing.
See text on page 145 for description.

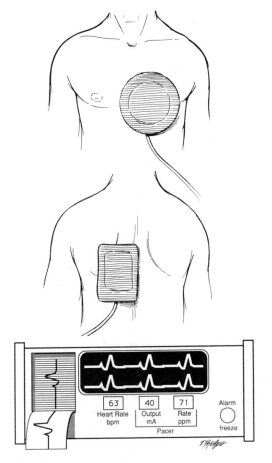

Figure 7-4. Transcutaneous pacing.
See text on page 146 for description.

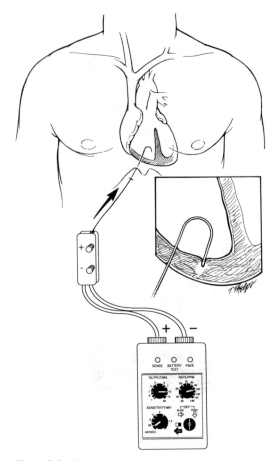

Figure 7-5. Transthoracic pacing.
See text on page 146 for description.

V. TACHYARRHYTHMIAS (Table 7-2)

A. Sinus Tachycardia (Figure 7-6A)

1. Characteristics
   The sinus rhythm exceeds 2 standard deviations of the resting mean heart rate for the patient's age (Table 1-1). Heart rates well in excess of 200 beats per minute can be seen as sinus tachycardia.

2. Etiology
   While these responses can be provoked by stress, attention should be given to analyzing the underlying conditions which include anemia, fever, hyperthyroidism, blood loss, and other physiologic disturbances.

3. Course
   In general, a documented sinus tachycardia should not be treated without first attempting correction of the underlying condition. Sinus tachycardia by itself is usually a benign rhythm in children except in the rare cases of coronary insufficiency (e.g., Kawasaki disease, anomalous left coronary artery, status post arterial switch procedure for transposition of the great arteries).

B. Supraventricular Tachycardia (SVT)
(Figure 7-6B and Table 7-2)

1. Characteristics
   The rate can vary from 150-350 beats per minute and in small infants there may be 1:1 conduction. The QRS is usually normal, although a right bundle branch block pattern may occur at fast rates. The p wave is usually not identifiable.

TABLE 7-2. Common Tachyarrhythmias

Rhythm	Rate		Characteristics		
	Atrial	Ventricular	Atrial Activity	Ventricular Activity	AV Conduction
Supraventricular tachycardia	150-350, regular	150-350, regular	Often not seen, or P wave may be in QRS or T	Normal or right bundle	1:1
Atrial flutter	250-350, regular	125-350, regular	Saw-tooth flutter waves in II, III, AVF	Normal	1:1, 2:1, or 3:1
Atrial fibrillation	300-600, irregular	100-350, irregular	Irregular fibrillation waves	Normal, bundle branch block, or bizarre	Varying
Ventricular tachycardia	Equals ventricular rate or less, regular	150-300, regular	Can be retrograde and inverted or normal	Bizarre, regular	1:1 retrograde or no relation
Ventricular fibrillation	---	100-300, irregular	---	Bizarre, irregular	---

2. Etiology

The etiology of this condition can be underlying heart disease such as Ebstein anomaly or Wolff-Parkinson-White syndrome. It can also occur in healthy children and can be provoked by physiologic stimulation since the rhythm involves a re-entry pathway which includes the AV node as well as the lower atrium. Many authorities consider atrial tachycardia, nodal tachycardia, and other names for fast supraventricular rates as varieties of SVT.

3. Course

This may result in heart failure in otherwise healthy children in whom fast rates are conducted to the ventricle.

4. Treatment

a. Vagal maneuvers
Enhanced vagal tone to slow conduction in the AV node often results in termination of arrhythmia. Application of ice to the face in infants and carotid massage in older children are useful techniques. Ocular compression should be avoided because it can result in permanent damage to the eye, including retinal detachment.

b. Pharmacotherapy (Table 7-3)
If vagal maneuvers are not effective, digitalis may be used both to convert the rhythm and for long term maintenance therapy. This is particularly useful in infants. Over one year of age, there is a choice of intravenous digoxin, verapamil, or

beta blockers. There is a particular concern in treatment of supraventricular arrhythmias due to Wolff-Parkinson-White syndrome, because digitalis and calcium blocking agents such as verapamil can speed up conduction over the accessory pathway and result in ventricular arrhythmias. Thus beta blockers or cardioversion may be preferred in Wolff-Parkinson-White syndrome.

TABLE 7-3. Pharmacotherapy of SVT

<u>Drug</u>	<u>Comments</u>
• phenylephrine (5-10 mg/kg)	• must raise BP by > 25%
• edrophonium (0.1 mg/kg)	• double dose until effect achieved; max (0.5 mg/kg)
• propranolol (begin with 0.5 mg)	• contraindicated if verapamil already given
• verapamil (0.1 mg/kg)	• contraindicated in infants

c. Cardioversion (Table 7-4)

Cardioversion is indicated in SVT with congestive heart failure or hypotension. Synchronized cardioversion is required in order to avoid the inadvertent development of ventricular fibrillation. (Instructions for cardioversion are listed in Table 7-4).

ERRATUM

GOLDEN HOUR:
THE HANDBOOK OF
ADVANCED PEDIATRIC
LIFE SUPPORT

by

David G. Nichols, M.D.
Myron Yaster, M.D.
Dorothy G. Lappe, R.N.
James R. Buck, M.D.

The dose of phenylephrine on
page 154, Table 7-3 should be
5-10 μg.

TABLE 7-4. Instructions for Cardioversion

1. Prep skin and apply electrodes
     White (RA)- near right midclavicular line, directly below clavicle.
     Black (LA)- near left midclavicular line, directly below clavicle.
     Red (LL)- Between 6th and 7th intercostal space on left midclavicular line
2. Connect cable to ECG input connector.
3. Turn defibrillator to monitor on position.
4. Display leads on machine.
5. Select SYNCHRONIZED mode on defibrillator.
6. Adjust ECG size until marker appears only with each R wave.
7. Select energy dosage: **0.25-0.5 J/kg**
8. Apply Electrode gel or defibrillator pads to paddles.
9. Apply paddles firmly to chest.
10. Press charge button.
11. Wait for charge to be completed.
12. Clear bed of contacts.
13. Press discharge buttons to deliver energy.

C. Atrial Flutter (Figure 7-6C)

1. Characteristics
   This classic rhythm is characterized by atrial rates which range from 250-400 beats/min and have characteristic saw-tooth flutter (F) waves on the ECG. These flutter waves are seen best in leads II, III, AVF, and V_1. In small infants there may be either 1:1 conduction or conduction block of 2:1 or 3:1. Sometimes this can be confused with supraventricular tachycardia when flutter waves may be seen before the QRS complex and missed during the QRS complex. QRS configurations are usually normal.

2. Etiology
   a. Atrial surgery (e.g., Fontan, Senning, or Mustard operations)
   b. Myocarditis
   c. Structural heart disease with dilated atria (e.g., Ebstein anomaly, tricuspid atresia, rheumatic mitral valve disease)

3. Course
   Congestive heart failure will develop if atrial flutter and rapid ventricular rates persist.

4. Treatment
   a. Cardioversion (Table 7-4)
      Synchronized cardioversion or overdrive pacing are useful therapies when rapid conversion is needed. Once cardioversion is obtained, it is possible to help prevent the recurrence of atrial flutter with a use of a wide variety of drugs including digoxin, quinidine or beta blockers.

   b. Pharmacotherapy (Table 7-5)
      Digitalis is used initially to slow the ventricular rate. Other, potentially useful, drugs such as quinidine and procainamide should be withheld until after digitalis is given, because these two drugs have the potential to produce vagolytic activity at relatively low doses. This may result in inadvertent increase in the ventricular rate and hemodynamic deterioration unless digitalis is given first.

D. Atrial Fibrillation (Figure 7-6D)

1. Characteristics

   The atrial activity is rapid and chaotic and the ventricular response can be irregular with a wide variety of ventricular rates. In the young patient who has not received digitalis, ventricular rates may be as high as 250 a minute, but they may be much slower (as low as 70 beats a minute) in a patient who is digitalized. The classic "irregularly irregular" pattern describes the ventricular response. The QRS form can vary since ventricular beats conducted rapidly after the preceding beat may have a right bundle branch block pattern while later beats may have a normal QRS configuration. The atrium may beat irregularly and the ventricular response may be regular when AV block occurs (e.g., digitalis effect) and the subsidiary nodal pace maker beats regularly.

2. Etiology

   Atrial fibrillation is seen most commonly with an enlarged atrium which can occur with rheumatic heart disease, particularly with rheumatic mitral valve disease. It can be seen in other conditions however such as with atrial septal defect, Ebstein anomaly, Wolff-Parkinson-White syndrome, or myocarditis. It is also to be suspected in patients who have left atrial volume overload such as is seen in patients with ventricular septal defects or after systemic to pulmonary artery palliative shunts.

3. Course
Atrial fibrillation is a sign of serious underlying heart disease which must be diagnosed and treated. Patients with marginal cardiac output may decompensate with the loss of coordinated atrial contraction during atrial fibrillation.

4. Treatment
   a. Cardioversion (Table 7-4)
   Cardioversion is usually effective in converting atrial fibrillation to sinus rhythm. However, signs of digitalis toxicity may become evident following conversion to a slow sinus rhythm in patients receiving high dose digitalis therapy for atrial fibrillation. Cardioversion may result in dislodgement of atrial clots with subsequent embolization in patients with longstanding atrial fibrillation, and anticoagulation of the patient should be considered before cardioversion is attempted.
   b. Pharmacotherapy
   The arrhythmia itself is generally effectively treated with digoxin which increases AV block and slows the ventricular rate. Patients with Wolff-Parkinson-White syndrome should not receive digoxin. Long term treatment to prevent recurrence often includes drugs such as quinidine or procainamide (Table 7-5).

E. Ventricular Tachycardia (Figure 7-6E)

1. Characteristics
The QRS complex is often wide and bizarre and is associated with a rapid rate of 150-250 beats per minute. Inversion of p waves which can be seen in at leads II, III, AVF suggests retrograde activation of the atria, and implies a diagnosis of ventricular

tachycardia. The differential diagnosis of ventricular tachycardia vs. supraventricular tachycardia with aberrancy is aided by the presence of a specific kind of ventricular fusion (Dressler) beat which is diagnostic of ventricular tachycardia. The ventricular fusion complex is produced by simultaneous capture of the ventricle with a supraventricular impulse and a ventricular impulse. The resultant fusion complex is intermediate in appearance between the normal supraventricular QRS configuration and the wide ventricular QRS configuration.

2. Etiology
This rhythm is generally seen in severe heart disease, drug ingestion, or in association with Wolff-Parkinson-White syndrome.

3. Course
Ventricular tachycardia is a life-threatening arrhythmia which demands immediate therapy.

4. Treatment
    a. Start CPR if no palpable pulse.
    b. Hypotensive patients should receive synchronized cardioversion.
    c. Normotensive patients with acute onset ventricular tachycardia receive pharmacotherapy starting with lidocaine 1 mg/kg IV. If lidocaine is unsuccessful, phenytoin 2-4 mg/kg IV over 5 min, propranolol 0.1 mg/kg IV slowly (max 1 mg), procainamide 2-6 mg/kg IV slowly, or bretylium 5 mg/kg IV slowly (for patients > 12 yrs) may be tried.

F. Ventricular Fibrillation (Figure 7-6F)

1. Characteristics
   This is an irregularly irregular rhythm in the ventricle which is associated with no cardiac output. The ventricular complexes can be fine or tall and undulating at rates of 100-300 a minute.

2. Etiology
   Ventricular fibrillation is a terminal rhythm which develops after hypoxia, ischemia, or following high voltage electrical injury. This rhythm is much less common in children than in adults who may develop ventricular fibrillation after myocardial infarction. Predisposing factors in children include Wolff-Parkinson-White and prolonged QT interval syndromes (Romano-Ward, Jervell-Lange-Nielson).

3. Course
   Cardiac arrest develops with the onset of ventricular fibrillation.

4. Treatment
   a. CPR
   b. Defibrillation 2 Joules/kg
   c. Epinephrine 0.1 mg/kg may turn fine fibrillation into course fibrillation and allow successful defibrillation.

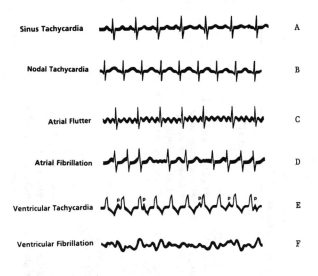

Figure 7-6. Tachyarrhythmias. (A) Sinus Tachycardia; (B) Supraventricular Tachycardia; (C) Atrial Flutter; (D) Atrial Fibrillation; (E) Ventricular Tachycardia; (F) Ventricular Fibrillation.

TABLE 7-5. Treatments Used in Cardiac Arrhythmias

NAME	DOSE	TOXICITY
Digoxin	<u>Total Digitalizing Dose (TDD)</u> • Total (give 75% if given IV) • Premature 0.02 mg/kg PO • Full-term 0.03 mg/kg PO • Under 2 yrs 0.04 mg/kg PO • Over 2 yrs 0.035 mg/kg PO • Maximum 1.0 mg PO • Give TDD as 3 doses over 24 hours (50%, 25%, 25%) <u>Maintenance</u> • Give 1/4 TDD in 2 divided doses (i.e., 1/8 TDD q 12h)	• 1°, 2°, 3° heart block • Other arrhythmias • Nausea, vomiting • Blurred vision • Increased toxicity with low potassium
Quinidine	<u>Oral Route Only</u> • 15-60 mg/kg 1 day • Give in 2-3 divided doses • Comes as sulfate or gluconate	• Increased QT • Increased QRS • Can increase AV conduction by vagolytic effect (See Atrial Flutter)

Procainamide

Intravenous
- Infants 7 mg/kg, give slowly (1 hour)
- Children 7-15 mg/kg, slowly (1 hour)

Oral
- 10-50 mg/kg/day given in split doses q 4-6 hr

- Can increase AV conduction (See Atrial Flutter)
- Induces Lupus Syndrome
- Can produce hypotension

Propranolol

Oral
- 1-3 mg/kg/day
- Divide into 4 doses

Intravenous
- Limit to 0.025 mg/kg
- Give over 20 minutes
- Do not repeat > 3 times

- Depressed myocardial contractility
- Interacts with Verapamil to profoundly depress myocardium.

Verapamil

Oral
- 4-15 mg/kg/day
- Divide into 3 doses
- Not with beta blockers

Intravenous
- 0.05-0.10 mg/kg to total 5 mg
- Can repeat 2-3 x with 15 minute interval

- Contraindicated < 1 year old can speed up WPW rhythms

Continued.

TABLE 7-5. (cont.).

<u>Amiodarone</u>	• 10 mg/kg/24h - q12h po x 7-10 days reduce to 5 mg/kg/24h if effective	• Use only in recurrent VT or other life-threatening circumstances • Slows AV conduction, Prolongs QRS • May depress myocardium
<u>Lidocaine</u>	• 1.0 mg/kg bolus • 10-50 ug/kg/min	• May produce pulmonary fibrosis • Relatively safe • Side effect is seizures
<u>Cardioversion</u>	<u>Synchronized</u> • 0.25-0.5 watt-sec/kg • Can increase to 1.0 watt-sec/kg if needed --- --- <u>Unsynchronized</u> • 2-6 watt-sec/kg	• Almost any cardiac rhythm requires synchronization except ventricular fibrillation. • Digitalis administration may be contraindication if patient heavily digitalized. • Reserved for ventricular fibrillation

Chapter 8
STATUS EPILEPTICUS

I. INTRODUCTION

A. Definition
Seizure activity lasting longer than 30 minutes.

B. Classification
The etiologies of status epilepticus are diverse (Table 8-1). In approximately **50% of patients**, status epilepticus is a **symptom** of an **underlying disease process**. In the remainder, the etiology of status epilepticus is either idiopathic epilepsy or febrile seizures.

TABLE 8-1. Status Epilepticus - Etiologies

Trauma	Metabolic disease
Neoplasms	Poisoning
Electrolyte disturbances	Hypoxic-ischemic injury
Cerebrovascular disease	Infection
Nutritional deficiencies	Cerebral malformations
Neurocutaneous syndromes	Degenerative brain diseases
Febrile seizures	Idiopathic epilepsy

II. PATHOPHYSIOLOGY OF BRAIN INJURY

A. Underlying disease
Injury caused by the underlying disease that precipitated the seizure, e.g., meningitis.

B. Systemic stress (especially hypoxia) resulting from obtundation, loss of airway protective reflexes, aspiration, etc. during repeated tonic-clonic seizures.

C. Direct injury caused by prolonged repetitive epileptic discharges.

III. MANAGEMENT

An aggressive and organized approach to management is necessary to prevent or minimize the morbidity and mortality resulting from status epilepticus. Management can be divided into three phases (Figure 8-1):

1. Emergency Stabilization

2. Anticonvulsant Therapy

3. Diagnostic Work-up

A. Emergency Stabilization (ABC's)

1. The primary goal of this phase is to prevent secondary hypoxic-ischemic brain injury.

2. Establish an adequate airway and ensure adequate oxygenation and ventilation. *Chapter 2* outlines Airway Management.

a. Suction oropharynx
b. Jaw thrust
c. 100% oxygen
d. Bag/mask ventilation (with cricoid pressure) if patient is cyanotic or ventilating inadequately (in preparation for intubation).
e. Intubation: usually requires the use of a muscle relaxant in addition to a sedative. A short acting agent (succinylcholine, 1.0 mg/kg or vecuronium, 0.1 mg/kg) should be used so that the presence of ongoing seizure activity can be assessed by physical examination after the effects of neuromuscular blockade have worn off.

3. Establish venous access and ensure adequate blood pressure.

a. Obtain blood for glucose determination (Chemstrip) and initial laboratory studies.
b. Administer 25% Dextrose 2.0 ml/kg IV if glucose is low.
c. If blood pressure is adequate, isotonic fluids should be given at minimum rates to minimize cerebral edema that may be present secondary to the patient's underlying disease process.

4. Assess the patient's cardiorespiratory status continuously during and after administration of anticonvulsants. (Respiratory depression and hypotension are common side effects.)

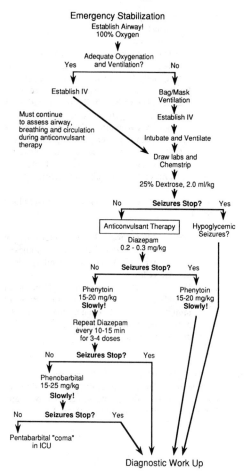

Figure 8-1. Approach to management of status epilepticus.

B. Anticonvulsant Therapy

1. Goals of this phase are twofold:

   a. Terminate seizure activity
   b. Prevent recurrences of seizure activity

2. Anticonvulsants (see Table 8-2).

   These agents should be administered intravenously. Absorption via intramuscular and rectal routes is too slow and too erratic for the treatment of status epilepticus.

   a. **Benzodiazepines** (diazepam and lorazepam) are widely used for acute control of seizures because of their extremely rapid onset of action. These drugs are not useful for long term prevention because of their short duration of action. Side effects of benzodiazepines include respiratory depression, sedation, and hypotension.

   b. **Phenytoin** is an effective agent for the treatment of status epilepticus, but has a relatively slow onset of action and is not an ideal agent for acute termination of seizure activity. It has two advantages over phenobarbital. First, phenytoin does not cause respiratory depression, and second, it causes much less sedation than phenobarbital. Side effects include bradycardia and hypotension. Phenytoin should be infused **slowly** ($<$ 50 mg/min for adults, 0.5-1 mg/kg/min for infants and children), and blood pressure and ECG should be monitored during the infusion.

c. **Phenobarbital**, like phenytoin, is an
effective anticonvulsant, but has a relatively
slow onset of action and is not an ideal
agent for acute termination of seizure
activity. Side effects include sedation,
respiratory depression, and hypotension.
Patients treated with a benzodiazepine
followed by a loading dose of phenobarbital
may require intubation because of
respiratory depression.

TABLE 8-2. Status Epilepticus - Anticonvulsants

Drug	Dosage	Onset	Duration
Diazepam	0.1-0.3 mg/kg/dose max = 10 mg/dose q 10-15 min	1-2 min	20-30 min
Lorazepam	0.05-0.1 mg/kg/dose max = 4 mg/dose q 10-15 min	2-10 min	> 3 hr
Phenytoin	loading dose 15-20 mg/kg give slowly! 0.5-1 mg/kg/min monitor ECG, BP	15-30 min	T 1/2 > 20 hr
Phenobarbital	loading dose 15-25 mg/kg give slowly!	20-30 min	T 1/2 > 20 hr

---

3. Strategy

There is no single therapeutic agent that will achieve both goals of this phase of management. Therefore, the clinician must use two drugs in the acute management of status epilepticus. One approach is to utilize a benzodiazepine for acute control followed by a loading dose of phenytoin to prevent recurrences:

a. **Step one**
Benzodiazepines should be given every 10-15 minutes until the seizure has been controlled.

b. **Step two**
A loading dose of phenytoin should be administered soon after the initial doses of benzodiazepine.

c. **Step three**
If seizures are not controlled after 3 doses of benzodiazepine and a loading dose of phenytoin, **a loading dose of phenobarbital** should be administered. Preparations should be made for intubation (respiratory depression is very likely in this setting).

d. **Step four**
General anesthesia with pentobarbital. If seizures do not respond to aggressive administration of benzodiazepines, phenytoin, and phenobarbital, general anesthesia with pentobarbital should be initiated **in an intensive care setting.**

e. Seizures secondary to underlying processes, e.g., hyponatremia, may be very difficult to control until precipitating factors have been identified and corrected (*Chapter 9*).

D. Diagnostic Work-up

1. Goals of this phase include diagnosing the underlying disease process and initiating definitive treatment.

2. After the patient is stabilized and seizures controlled, an exhaustive history and physical examination should be performed.

3. Laboratory evaluation
   CBC, electrolytes, glucose, calcium, magnesium, phosphate, BUN, creatinine, urinalysis, blood culture, toxicology screen, ammonia, metabolic screen for inborn error of metabolism (infants), and anticonvulsant levels (for patients on chronic anticonvulsants).

4. Indications for computed tomography and lumbar puncture are summarized in Tables 8-3 and 8-4, respectively. It is imperative that the patient be stabilized **prior** to CT scan and lumbar puncture.

TABLE 8-3.   **Status Epilepticus - Indications For Emergency Computed Tomography**

- Head trauma
- Physical exam suggestive of increased intracranial pressure
- Focal neurological deficit
- Focal seizure activity

TABLE 8-4. Status Epilepticus - Indications and Contraindications for Lumbar Puncture

---

Indications

- Presence of meningeal signs

- Febrile child less than 18 months of age

- Immunocompromised host

Contraindications

- Severe coagulopathy, thrombocytopenia

- Cardiopulmonary instability

- Evidence of increased intracranial pressure

- Focal seizures or focal neurological deficit (unless normal CT)

- Infection at site of needle insertion

Chapter 9
NONTRAUMATIC STUPOR
AND COMA

I. INTRODUCTION

A. Classification

1. **Stupor** is a state of unresponsiveness from which the patient can be aroused by vigorous stimulation. The stuporous patient will lapse back into the unresponsive state when the stimulus is withdrawn.

2. **Coma** is a state of unresponsiveness from which the patient cannot be aroused.

B. Altered states of consciousness can result from a vast number of disease processes (Table 9-1).

C. In the acute care setting, the clinician must remember that any acute alteration of consciousness represents significant neurologic dysfunction and must be regarded as a life-threatening emergency.

II. PATHOPHYSIOLOGY

A. Conscious behavior requires intact function of the brainstem reticular activating system and both cerebral hemispheres.

B. Stupor or coma results from dysfunction or destruction of either the ascending reticular activating system or both cerebral hemispheres. Unilateral injury or dysfunction of the cerebral hemispheres will not cause stupor or coma unless the injury produces secondary effects, e.g., ischemia, upon the contralateral hemisphere.

C. **Stupor and coma** are signs of "brain failure" and must be treated emergently in an effort to prevent or minimize irreversible central nervous system injury.

TABLE 9-1. Common Causes of Coma in Infants and Children

Trauma	Cerebrovascular disease
Poisoning	Obstructive hydrocephalus
Hypernatremia	Seizures and post-ictal states
Hyperammonemia	Hypoxic-ischemic brain injury
Infection	Uremia
Hypercapnia	Diabetic ketoacidosis
Hypoglycemia	Hypothermia

III. MANAGEMENT

A. **Goals of management** are three-fold.

1. Prevent secondary hypoxic-ischemic brain injury.

2. Prevent herniation.

3. Diagnose and treat (if possible) the underlying cause of coma.

B. Classification of Causes of Coma

This very simple classification scheme establishes priorities for both diagnosis and treatment and provides the framework upon which this management approach (Figure 9-1) is based.

Dean JM, Hanley DF. Evaluation of the comatose child. In **Textbook of Pediatric Intensive Care**, Rogers MC (ed), Williams & Wilkins, Baltimore, MD, 1987.

1. **Immediately Treatable Metabolic Coma**

   a. Hypoglycemia
   b. Meningitis
   c. Opioid overdose (poisoning)

2. **Rapidly Progressive Intracranial Lesions**

   a. Trauma
   b. Cerebrovascular disease
   c. Infection
   d. Malignancy
   e. Hydrocephalus

3. **Stable Coma**

   a. All causes of coma except hypoglycemia, meningitis, and intracranial mass lesions
   b. "Stable" only if the patient is receiving adequate cardiorespiratory support.

C. Management

1. Emergency Stabilization

2. Diagnostic Work-up

3. Definitive Treatment

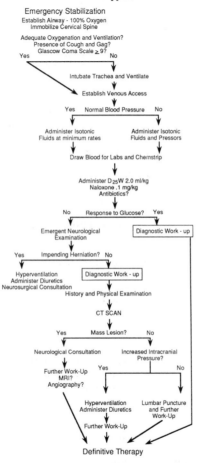

Figure 9-1. Management of coma.

D. Emergency Stabilization - ABC's

1. This phase begins upon arrival of the patient and continues during the diagnostic work-up and definitive treatment phases.

2. Goals of this phase of management are two-fold.
   a. Prevent secondary hypoxic-ischemic brain injury
   b. Prevent herniation

3. Establish an adequate airway and ensure adequate oxygenation and ventilation (*Chapter 2*).
   a. All comatose patients should have their cervical spine immobilized until spinal injury has been ruled out.
   b. 100% oxygen
   c. Jaw thrust
   d. Oral airway
   e. Indications for intubation (Table 9-2.)

TABLE 9-2. Indications for Intubation of the Comatose Child

- Inability to maintain patent airway
- Glasgow Coma Scale < 8 (Table 9-3)
- Absent cough
- Absent gag
- Hypoxemia
- Hypoventilation
- Impending herniation (hyperventilation Rx)

TABLE 9-3. Glasgow Coma Scale

Response	Adults & Children	Infants	Points
Eye Opening	no response	no response	1
	to pain	to pain	2
	to voice	to voice	3
	spontaneous	spontaneous	4
Verbal	no response	no response	1
	incomprehensible	moans to pain	2
	inappropriate words	cries to pain	3
	disoriented conversation	irritable	4
	oriented and appropriate	coos, babbles	5
Motor	no response	no response	1
	decerebrate posturing	decerebrate posturing	2
	decorticate posturing	decorticate posturing	3
	withdraws to pain	withdraws to pain	4
	localizes pain	withdraws to touch	5
	obeys commands	normal spontaneous movement	6
Total Score			3-15

4. Establish venous access and ensure an adequate blood pressure (*Chapter 6*).

   a. If the patient is hypotensive, isotonic fluids and vasopressors should be administered as necessary to maintain a normal blood pressure.

b. If the patient is normotensive, isotonic fluids should be administered at the lowest possible rates to minimize cerebral edema that may be present secondary to the patient's underlying disease.

c. Blood should be obtained for glucose determination and initial laboratory studies.

d. Dextrose, 25%, 2.0 ml/kg, should be administered. **(Immediately Treatable Metabolic Coma)**

e. If patient has fever and meningismus, antibiotics should be administered after obtaining a blood culture (*Chapter 12*) **(Immediately Treatable Metabolic Coma)**.

f. Although narcotic overdose is extremely rare in children, naloxone, 0.1 mg/kg, may be administered at this time.

5. Perform emergent neurological examination to assess for impending herniation.
   a. Level of consciousness - Glasgow Coma Scale (Table 9-3)
   b. Extraocular movements
      (1) Oculocephalic reflex (doll's eyes)
      (2) Oculovestibular reflex (cold calorics)
   c. Pupillary response to light

6. Signs suggestive of impending herniation (Figure 9-2):
   a. Asymmetric motor response to pain.
   b. Decorticate or decerebrate responses to pain
   c. Cranial nerve palsies (especially unilateral or bilateral fixed pupils).
   d. Cushing's triad (irregular respiration, hypertension, and bradycardia).
   e. Other abnormalities of vital signs (tachycardia, hypertension, or hypotension).

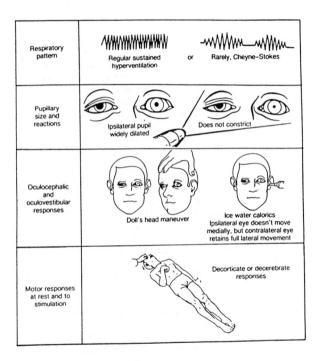

Figure 9-2. Signs of impending herniation.
From Plum F, Posner JB. **The Diagnosis of Stupor and Coma.**
Third Edition. Philadelphia, PA, FA Davis, 1982, p 104, 111.

7. Treat impending herniation.
    a. Hyperventilation is the primary mode of therapy. Titrate to signs of impending herniation, e.g., a fixed and dilated pupil becomes smaller and reacts to light during hyperventilation.
    b. Diuretics (furosemide 1.0 mg/kg or mannitol 0.25 gm/kg) can also be administered at this time provided blood pressure is stable. Diuretics have a delayed effect and should never be used in lieu of hyperventilation for impending herniation.
    c. Obtain neurosurgical consultation
    d. Emergent CT scan to rule out a mass lesion. **(Rapidly Progressive Intracranial Lesions)**

E. Diagnostic Work-up

1. This phase begins upon arrival of the patient but becomes a major priority only after the patient has been stabilized and immediately life-threatening causes of coma **(Immediately Treatable Metabolic Coma and Rapidly Progressive Intracranial Lesions)** have been appropriately treated.
2. If the clinician feels the patient is **not** at risk of impending herniation, a history and physical examination may be performed while preparations are being made for CT scanning.
3. Computed tomography will determine if a mass lesion is present. If present, neurosurgical consultation should be obtained. If no mass lesion is identified, then the clinician can proceed with an exhaustive work-up to determine the etiology of coma **(Stable Coma)**. A detailed physical examination should be the first step in this process.

4. Initial laboratory evaluation should include arterial blood gas, carboxyhemoglobin, CBC, electrolytes, osmolality, glucose, calcium, magnesium, phosphate, ammonia, coagulation studies, BUN, creatinine, blood culture, toxicology screen, urinalysis, and urine culture.

5. A lumbar puncture may be performed only after the patient has been stabilized and there are no other contraindications (mass lesion, increased intracranial pressure, coagulopathy, focal neurologic deficit, infection at site of puncture).

6. History and physical exam will guide the clinician for further diagnostic studies.

F. Definitive Therapy

Once the diagnosis has been established, definitive therapy may be initiated.

IV. DIABETIC KETOACIDOSIS (DKA)

A. Definition

Hyperglycemia (glucose > 300 mg/dl), ketonemia (ketones present at > 1:2 dilution), acidosis (pH < 7.3 or HCO_3^- < 15 mEq/L), ketonuria, and glucosuria define DKA in the patient with a history compatible with diabetes mellitus.

B. Pathophysiology

1. Diabetes mellitus arises from inadequate amounts of insulin. The absence of insulin results in:
   a. Increased
      (1) glycogenolysis
      (2) gluconeogenesis
      (3) proteolysis
      (4) lipolysis
      (5) ketogenesis

      b.   Decreased
          (1)   glucose utilization
          (2)   ketone utilization

2.   The resultant hyperglycemia and hyperketonemia produce an osmotic diuresis (water, sodium, potassium, phosphate, calcium), dehydration, metabolic (lactic) acidosis, and hypotension. Diabetic coma correlates with serum osmolality. The patient's clouded sensorium usually clears as the hyperosmolar state is corrected.

C. Fluid and Electrolyte Changes

1.   Serum Osmolality (mOsm/L) =
$$2 \times Na + \frac{glucose\ (mg/dl)}{18} + \frac{BUN\ (mg/dl)}{2.8}$$

2.   Dehydration (10-15% of body weight)

3.   Factitious hyponatremia is often reported secondary to severe lipemia (Na ↓ by 0.002 x lipid mg/dl). Serum sodium decreases by 1.6 mEq/L for each 100 mg/dl rise in glucose.

4.   Hyperchloremia may arise during fluid replacement therapy with normal saline.

5.   Potassium
      a.   Severe total body potassium depletion is common even when serum levels are normal initially. Serum levels will drop with administration of insulin.

6.   Hypophosphatemia
      a.   Depresses red blood cell 2,3-diphosphoglycerate.
      b.   Results in muscle weakness and easy fatiguability.

D. Management

1. Fluids
   a. Assume 10-15% dehydration. Ringer's lactate (RL) or normal saline, 10-20 ml/kg over 1 hour. If in shock, administer RL as rapidly and as possible until perfusion returns to normal.
   b. First 8 hours: 0.45 NS + 40 mEq/L of [K$^+$], 1/2 as KCl, 1/2 as KPO$_4$. Do not give potassium, if [K$^+$] is elevated or if the patient is not urinating. Replace 1/2 of the remaining deficit + insensible losses + urine output (which may be enormous 2° to osmotic diuresis). KPO$_4$ administration may produce hypocalcemic tetany.
   c. Next 16-24 hours: replace the remainder of the deficit + maintenance requirements (*Chapter 5*). Urine output should decrease as hyperglycemia is corrected.
   d. If the initial pH is < 7.10 or [HCO$_3$] is < 5 mEq/L, consider adding 10-40 mEq/L bicarbonate to the initial IV solution.

2. Insulin
   a. IV infusion is the preferred technique. There is less risk of a precipitous fall in glucose and serum osmoles, thereby potentially reducing the risk of cerebral edema.
   b. Give 0.1 units/kg of regular insulin as an IV bolus, then 0.1 units/kg/hr.
   c. Increase insulin up to 0.2 units/kg/hr if glucose falls at < 50 mg/dl/hr.
   d. If glucose falls > 100 mg/dl/hr or if the patient remains ketotic, continue insulin at 0.1 units/kg/hr but add glucose to the IV solution.

3. Glucose
    a. Measure serum glucose hourly. The rate of glucose fall should not exceed 100 mg/dl/hour.
    b. As glucose approaches 300 mg/dl add glucose to the IV solution.
4. Ketosis
    a. Ketosis often fails to resolve if:
        (1) infection is present
        (2) fluids are inadequately replaced

E. Monitoring

1. Every 1-2 hours
   Vital signs, glucose determination
2. Every 3-4 hours
   Glucose, pH, PCO_2, electrolytes, calcium, phosphate

F. Progressive Cerebral Edema 2° to Therapy

Rarely, the treatment of DKA is accompanied by progressive deepening coma, increased intracranial pressure, and even death. This may be associated with bicarbonate therapy and too rapid correction of serum hyperosmolality. Lumbar puncture is contraindicated in this situation.

V. HYPERNATREMIA

A. Etiology of Hypernatremia Dehydration

Hypernatremia may be caused by excessive water loss (diabetes insipidus, nephropathy, diarrhea) or salt poisoning (boiled skim milk, mineralocorticoid excess).

B. Treatment of Hypernatremia

1. Free water deficit is **ESTIMATED** to be 4ml/kg for every mEq that the serum sodium exceeds 145 mEq/L.

2. The degree of dehydration is difficult to assess, because circulating volume is relatively preserved at the expense of cellular water.

3. Replace fluids **slowly** over 48-72 hours. More rapid corrections can cause cerebral edema and seizures.

4. First hour
   Resuscitate with 10-20 ml/kg of Lactated Ringer's solution to expand the extra-cellular fluid volume and perfuse the kidneys.

5. Hours 2-72
   Calculate maintenance and deficit fluid and replace with $D_5.45NaCl$.

6. In salt poisoning (exogenous sodium, boiled skim milk) consider peritoneal dialysis.

7. In diabetes insipidus, start Vasopressin infusion at 0.005 units/kg/hr.

8. Slow rehydration is the rule.

VI. OBSTRUCTED VENTRICULAR SHUNTS

A child with a malfunctioning ventricular shunt is evaluated according to the scheme in Table 9-4.

A. Shunt Obstruction with Mild Symptoms (vomiting and stupor)

1. Observe ABC's.
2. Urgent neurosurgical consultation.
3. CT scan.

B. Shunt Obstruction with Impending Herniation

1. Observe ABC's.
2. Urgent neurosurgical consultation. If no neurosurgeon is immediately available, proceed with shunt aspiration.
3. Aspiration of cerebral spinal fluid (CSF) from the proximal shunt chamber.
   a. Wash skin with 10% iodine solution and allow to dry.
   b. Insert 25 gauge butterfly needle attached to a stopcock and 10 cc syringe into the proximal shunt chamber and remove sufficient fluid to relieve symptoms.
   c. Send CSF sample for gram stain, cell count, glucose, protein, and culture.

TABLE 9-4. Management of Obstructed Ventricular Shunts

Status of Patient	Status of Shunt	Probable Diagnosis	Solution
normal	pumps freely fills freely	functional shunt	routine follow up
	pumps freely fills slowly	partial obstruction ventricular end -plugged with choroid plexus or ependyma -ventricle collapses on shunt tip	close follow up
normal	pumps with difficulty or not at all	-obstructed distal end; probable dx: compensated hydrocephalus	close follow up
symptomatic	pumps freely fills freely	-disconnection in shunt system -cyst around peritoneal end -symptoms may not be shunt related	-repair shunt -revise distal end -diagnostic tests
symptomatic	pumps freely, refills slowly or not at all	-obstructed ventricular end	revise shunt emergently, tap shunt
symptomatic	pumps poorly or not at all	-distal obstruction resulting from growth of patient, kinking of tubing, clot, adhesions	revise shunt emergently, tap shunt

Chapter 10
PAIN CONTROL AND SEDATION

I. OVERVIEW

Even when their pain is obvious, children frequently receive inadequate or no treatment for pain. The common "wisdom", that children neither respond to, nor remember, painful experiences to the same degree that adults do, is simply not true. In order to achieve satisfactory sedation and analgesia, various drugs, administered alone and in combination, can be safely given to children by various routes.

II. PAIN ASSESSMENT

Pain is a subjective experience and can be defined operationally as "what the patient says hurts" and exists "when the patient says it does." In order to effectively treat pain one must be able to accurately measure it. In children older than 3 years of age we use visual analogue scales (Figure 10-1) either:

      1) a 10 cm line with a smiling face at one end and a
         distraught crying face at the other, (Figure 10-1)
      2) a 9 face interval scale

Alternatively, in older children, we suggest using numerical rating scales in which 0 is no pain and 10 the worst pain the child has ever experienced.

III. PATIENT MONITORING (Table 10-1)

When administering potent analgesics, the physician must anticipate, recognize and be able to treat potentially life-threatening adverse drug effects. Compulsive monitoring is required not only during the administration of these drugs and during the performance of a procedure but extends until a patient awakens.

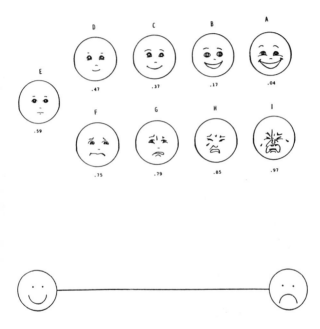

Figure 10-1. Pain assessment (visual analogue) scales.
The higher the score, the greater the child's pain. The 9 face interval scale was developed by Dr. James W. Varni and is reprinted with permission. The 10 centimeter linear analogue scale is reproduced with permission from Dr. Patricia A. McGrath.

TABLE 10-1.   Emergency Drugs and Equipment Required for Sedation and Local Anesthetic Administration

Personnel for procedures
- The practitioner performing the procedure
- A **2nd** person, qualified to monitor and administer drugs, who is **NOT** performing the procedure:

Equipment for intravenous access
- Catheters (various sizes), administration sets
- Fluids (Ringer's Lactate, D_5W + salt (0.2, 0.45, 0.9%), albumen)

Emergency cart
- Suction (large bore device, e.g., Yankauer)
- Oxygen and oxygen delivery system
- Airway
    1) oral airways (various sizes)
    2) masks (various sizes)
    3) laryngoscope and appropriate size blades
    4) endotracheal tubes (various sizes)
    5) stylet

Drugs
    1) Epinephrine
    2) Bicarbonate
    3) Atropine
    4) Lidocaine, bretylium
    5) Glucose
    6) Naloxone, physostigmine
    7) Anticonvulsants (thiopental, diazepam or midazolam)

Monitoring equipment (should be used in all children in whom consciousness may be lost)
- Pulse oximeter
- Blood pressure
- ECG

IV. OPIOID ANALGESICS (Table 10-3)

At equianalgesic doses all commonly used opioids produce similar degrees of respiratory depression, hemodynamic collapse, euphoria, sedation, nausea, biliary tract spasm, and constipation.

A. Risk Factors when Prescribing Opioids or Sedative/Hypnotics (Table 10-2)

1. Adverse cardio-respiratory effects associated with opioid or sedative/hypnotics administration depend on:
   a. dose
   b. rate of drug administration
   c. concomitant administration of other drugs
   d. patient's age and medical history

TABLE 10-2. **Medical Conditions Associated with Increased Risk of Cardiorespiratory Complications Following Opioid or Sedative Administration**

- Infants < 3 months of age
- Premature infants < 60 post-conceptual weeks of age
- History of apnea or disordered control of breathing
- Cardio-respiratory disease
- Hemodynamic instability
- Obtundation
- Airway compromise

---

2. The combination of an opioid and a sedative significantly increases the risk of respiratory depression. In fact, it is often necessary to reduce the dose of both families of drugs to levels below that generally recommended for either drug when used by itself.

TABLE 10-3. Commonly used opioids*			
Name	Equipotent dose (mg/kg)	Duration (h)	Comments
Morphine	0.1	3-4	1) vasodilator, avoid in shock and hemodynamically unstable patient 2) seizures in high doses and in newborn 3) releases histamine
Fentanyl	0.001	0.5-1	1) bradycardia 2) chest wall rigidity, treated with naloxone 3) IV route only
Meperidine	1.0	3-4	1) catastrophic interactions with MAO inhibitors 2) toxic metabolite 3) tachycardia
Codeine	1.2	3-4	1) best prescribed with acetaminophen 2) PO only
Methadone	0.1	4-12	1) can be given IV, IM or PO; oral bioavailability 100%

* Opioid dosages must be individualized and administered by titration to effect, rather than by a fixed dosage schedule, formulated by weight.

IV= intravenous, IM= intramuscular, PR=rectal, PO= oral

B. Opioid Antagonists (Naloxone) (Table 10-4)

Naloxone is extremely potent and non-selective in its ability to antagonize opioid effects. It antagonizes not only the respiratory depression, chest wall rigidity, sedation and gastrointestinal effects of the opioids but the analgesia as well. Great caution must be exercised in antagonizing opioids in patients who are chronically dependent on opioids or who are in severe pain. It is our practice to mechanically ventilate these patients as an alternative.

Naloxone is supplied as a parenteral solution (0.4 mg/ml and 0.02 mg/ml). It can be administered intravenously or intramuscularly.

TABLE 10-4. Indications for Naloxone Use

Problem	Dose (mg/kg)
Itching, urinary retention	0.001-0.002
Biliary spasm	0.001-0.002
Respiratory depression in an opioid dependent patient or a patient in severe pain	0.001, increase in a step-wise fashion: 0.002, 0.004, 0.006, etc.; or mechanical ventilation
Overdose	0.01-0.1
Newborn (maternal opioids)	0.01-1.0

The plasma elimination half life of naloxone is 60 minutes which is significantly shorter than the opioids it is being used to antagonize. Thus, patients may require repeat intravenous doses, intramuscular (depot) injections, or continuous infusions. Patients must be monitored for possible return of respiratory depression following naloxone treatment. At a minimum, this requires pulse oximetry and clinical observation.

V. LOCAL ANESTHETICS (Table 10-5)

The administration of local anesthetics ("regional" blockade) is an effective, safe, and easy method of providing pain relief, particularly for "procedure related" pain and for post-traumatic pain (e.g., fractures).

A. Drug Dosage and Toxicity

Toxicity to local anesthetics is determined by the total dose of drug administered and by the rapidity of absorption into the blood. The newborn may be particularly vulnerable. A continuum of toxic effects exists:

1. Mild: tinnitus, light-headedness, visual and auditory disturbances, restlessness, muscular twitching
2. Severe: seizures, arrhythmias, coma, cardiovascular collapse, respiratory arrest

B. Subcutaneous Infiltration

1. To minimize the pain of injection
   a. use either 25 or 26 gauge needles
   b. add bicarbonate to the local anesthetic (9 ml local anesthetic + 1 ml bicarbonate)
   c. inject as the needle is being advanced

C. Peripheral Nerve Blocks (Figure 10-2, 10-3)

1. Epinephrine is added to local anesthetics to increase the duration and intensity of a block. **Never inject epinephrine-containing solutions into areas supplied by end-arteries, such as the digits.**
2. Increased concentration of local anesthetic increases the incidence of motor blockade and toxicity. It affects sensory blockade only minimally.

TABLE 10-5. Maximum Dosage of Local Anesthetic Agents for Peripheral Nerve or Subcutaneous Infiltration*	
Drug (Concentration)	**Dose (mg/kg)**
Lidocaine (Xylocaine®)(0.5-2.0%)	7-10†
Bupivacaine (Marcaine®) (0.25-0.50%)	2-3†
Tetracaine (Pontocaine®) (0.1-0.2%)	2
Procaine (Novocain®) (0.5-10%)	10-15†
Prilocaine (Citanest®) (1-2%)	5-7‡‡

*   These are suggested safe upper limits for local anesthetic administration.   Accidental intravenous or intra-arterial injection of even a fraction of these amounts may result in systemic toxicity.

†   The higher dose is recommended only with the concomitant use of epinephrine 1:200,000

For topical intranasal use only, maximum dose 200 mg

‡‡   Maximum dose 600 mg, is not recommended in children less than 6 months of age

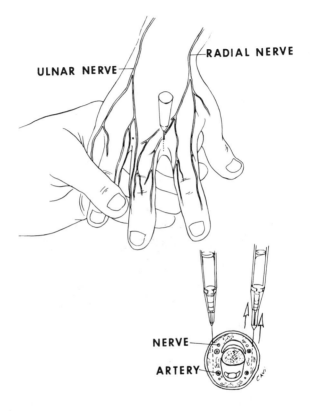

Figure 10-2. Digital nerve block.
Insert 25 gauge needle between the heads of the metacarpals (-tarsals) on either side of the digit. Inject 1-3 ml of local anesthetic continuously while advancing the needle from the dorsal to the volar surface of the digit.

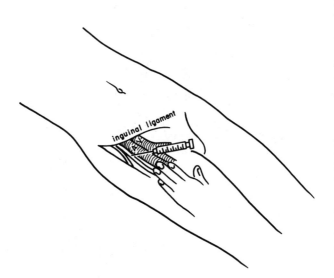

Figure 10-3. Femoral nerve block.
The femoral artery is compressed against the underlying bone. A 22-
or 25 gauge needle is inserted perpendicularly, approximately 1/2 to
1 cm lateral to the pulsation of the femoral artery (A) and 3-10 ml of
local anesthetic is injected following a negative aspiration of blood.

Chapter 11
DRUG INTOXICATION

I. EPIDEMIOLOGY

Eighty-five to ninety percent of pediatric poisoning occurs in children less than 5 years of age and is accidental. Poisoning in older children accounts for the remaining 10-15% and is generally considered intentional.

II. DIAGNOSIS OF POISONING

Tables 11-1 through 11-4 describe the general presentation, clinical clues, toxidromes and pertinent laboratory data which are useful in the diagnosis of poisoning.

TABLE 11-1. General Presentations Suggestive of Poisoning

• Acutely disturbed consciousness	• Arrhythmias
• Abnormal behavior	• Metabolic acidosis
• Seizures	• Severe vomiting, diarrhea
• Unusual odor	• Cyanosis
• Shock	• Respiratory distress

III. TREATMENT

A. Resuscitation and Stabilization

Ensure adequate airway, breathing, circulation and seizure control before diagnostic steps or specific antidotal therapy is instituted. Respiratory failure, hypotension, arrhythmias and seizures are the most life-threatening systemic complications of drug intoxication.

TABLE 11-2.   Clinical Clues to the Diagnosis of the Unknown Poison

	Sign or Symptom	Poison
Odor		
	Bitter almond	Cyanide
	Acetone	Isopropyl alcohol, methanol, acetylsalicylic acid
	Pungent aromatic	Ethchlorvynol
	Oil of wintergreen	Methyl salicylate
	Garlic	Arsenic, phosphorus, thallium, organophosphates
	Alcohol	Ethanol, methanol
	Petroleum	Petroleum distillates
Skin		
	Cyanosis	Methemoglobinemia secondary to nitrates, nitrites, phenacetin, benzocaine
	Red flush	Carbon monoxide, cyanide, boric acid, anticholinergics
	Sweating	Amphetamines, LSD, organophosphates, cocaine, barbiturates
	Dry	Anticholinergics
Temperature		
	Hypothermia	Sedative hypnotics, ethanol, carbon monoxide, phenothiazines, tricyclic antidepressants (TCA), clonidine
	Hyperthermia	Anticholinergics, salicylates, phenothiazines, TCA, cocaine, amphetamines, theophylline

Blood pressure

      Hypertension   Sympathomimetics (especially phenylpropanolamine in over-the-counter cold remedies), organophosphates, amphetamine, phencyclidine, cocaine

Pulse Rate

      Bradycardia   Digitalis, sedative hypnotics, beta blockers, ethchlorvynol, narcotics

      Tachycardia   Anticholinergics, sympathomimetics, amphetamine, alcohol, aspirin, theophylline, cocaine, TCA

      Arrhythmias   Anticholinergics, TCA, organophosphates, phenothiazines, digoxin, beta-blockers, carbon monoxide, cyanide

Mucous Membranes

      Dry   Anticholinergics

      Salivation   Organophosphates, carbamates

      Oral lesions   Corrosives, paraquat

      Lacrimation   Caustics, organophosphates, irritant gases

Respiration

      Depressed   Alcohol, narcotics, barbiturates, sedative/hypnotics

      Tachypnea   Salicylates, amphetamines, carbon monoxide

      Kussmaul   Methanol, ethylene glycol, salicylates

      Wheezing   Organophosphates

      Pneumonia   Hydrocarbons

Continued.

TABLE 11-2. (cont.).

Pulmonary edema	Aspiration, salicylates, narcotics, sympathomimetics
Central Nervous System	
Seizures	Camphor, carbon monoxide, cocaine, amphetamines and sympathomimetics, anticholinergics, aspirin, pesticides organophosphates, PCP, phenothiazines, lead, isoniazid, lithium, strychnine
Miosis	Narcotics (except Meperidine and Lomotil), phenothiazines, organophosphates (late), benzodiazepines, barbiturates, mushrooms (muscarine types), barbiturates (late)
Mydriasis	Anticholinergics, sympathomimetics (cocaine, amphetamines, LSD, PCP), TCA, methanol, glutethimide
Blindness, optic atrophy	Methanol
Fasciculation	Organophosphates
Nystagmus	Diphenylhydantoin, barbiturates, carbamazepine, PCP, carbon monoxide, glutethimide, ethanol

Hypertonus	Anticholinergics, strychnine, phenothiazines
Myoclonus, rigidity	Anticholinergics, phenothiazines, haloperidol
Delirium/psychosis	Anticholinergics, sympathomimetics, alcohol, phenothiazines, PCP, LSD, marijuana, cocaine, heroin, methaqualone, heavy metals
Coma	Alcohols, anticholinergics, sedative hypnotics, narcotics, carbon monoxide, tricyclic antidepressants, salicylates, organophosphates
Weakness, paralysis	Organophosphates, carbamates, heavy metals

Gastrointestinal System

Vomiting, diarrhea	Iron, phosphorus, heavy metals, lithium, mushrooms, fluoride, organophosphates

Adapted from: Mofenson NC, Greensher J: The unknown poison. Pediatrics 54: 337, 1974. Reproduced with permission.

TABLE 11-3. Toxidromes

Drug Involved	Clinical Manifestations
Anticholinergics (atropine, scopolamine, tricyclic antidepressants, antihistamines, mushrooms)	Agitation, hallucinations, coma, extrapyramidal movements, mydriasis. Flushed, warm, dry skin; dry mouth. Tachycardia, arrythmias, hypotension, hypertension. Decreased bowel sounds.
Cholinergics (organophosphate and carbamate insecticides)	Salivation, lacrimation, urination, defecation, nausea, vomiting, sweating. Bronchorrhea, rales and wheezes. Weakness, paralysis, confusion, coma, muscle fasciculations and miosis.
Opiates	Bradycardia, hypotension. Pulmonary edema, slow respirations. Seizures, hypothermia, coma, miosis.
Sedative/Hypnotics	Coma, hypothermia. Slow respirations. Hypotension, tachycardia.
Tricyclic Antidepressants	Coma, convulsions, arrhythmias, anticholinergic manifestations.
Salicylates	Vomiting, hyperpnea, fever, lethargy, coma.

Phenothiazines	Hypotension, tachycardia, torsion of head and neck, oculogyric crisis, trismus, ataxia, anticholinergic manifestations.
Sympathomimetics (amphetamines, phenylpropanolamine, ephedrine, caffeine, cocaine, aminophylline)	Tachycardia, arrhythmias. Psychosis, hallucinations, delirium. Nausea, vomiting, abdominal pain, piloerection.
Alcohol, isopropanol, methanol, ethylene, glycol, salicylates, paraldehyde, toluene	Elevated anion gap metabolic acidosis.

Adapted from: Mofenson NC, Greensher J: The unknown poison. Pediatrics 54:337, 1974.

TABLE 11-4. Routine Laboratory Tests That Can Suggest Poisoning

Test	Poisons
• Decreased hemoglobin saturation with normal or increased PO$_2$	• Agents causing methemoglobinemia (nitrates, nitrites, benzocaine)
• Elevated anion gap metabolic acidosis*	• Methanol, ethanol, isopropyl alcohol, ethylene glycol, salicylates, isoniazid, paraldehyde, toluene, iron, phenformin, carbon monoxide, cyanide
• Elevated osmolar gap**	• Ethanol, methanol, isopropyl alcohol, ethylene glycol
• Hypoglycemia	• Insulin, ethanol, isopropyl alcohol, isoniazid, acetaminophen, salicylates, oral hypoglycemic agents
• Hyperglycemia	• Salicylates, isoniazid, organophosphates, iron
• Hypocalcemia	• Ethylene glycol, methanol
• Urinalysis	
Oxalic acid crystalluria	• Ethylene glycol
Ketonuria	• Isopropyl alcohol, ethanol, salicylates

* Anion gap = Na - (Cl + HCO$_3$) Normal value 8-12 mEq/l
** Osmolar gap = measured osmolality - calculated osmolality
Calculated osmolality = (2 x Na) + (BUN/2.8) + (glucose/18).

From: Berkowitz ID, Rogers MC: Poisoning and the critically ill child. In Rogers MC (ed) **Textbook of Pediatric Intensive Care.** Williams and Wilkins, Baltimore 1987.

B. Prevention of Further Drug Absorption

1. Surface decontamination of external poisons
   a. Skin
      Remove clothes, wash skin (e.g., for organophosphates).
   b. Eyes
      Copious irrigation (e.g., for liquid corrosives).

C. Gastrointestinal Tract Decontamination (Table 11-5)

1. Emesis, lavage
   Because many drugs delay gastric emptying, emesis or lavage must be performed irrespective of the time elapsed since ingestion.
2. Activated charcoal
   This effectively absorbs many different drugs, thereby decreasing systemic absorption.
3. Cathartics
   Cathartics are administered in oral intoxications to decrease drug absorption by shortening gastrointestinal transit time.

D. Hastening Elimination of Poisons from Blood and Tissues

1. Forced diuresis with/without alteration of pH
   Alkaline diuresis can be achieved by administration of 2-5 times maintenance fluid requirements to achieve urine flow of 2-5 ml/kg/hr. Add $NaHCO_3$ 50-75 mEq/L and KCl 40-60 mEq/L of IV fluid to achieve urine pH >7.5. Follow serum K^+ to avoid hypokalemia. Contraindications include cerebral and pulmonary edema and renal failure.
2. Dialysis (Table 11-6)
3. Hemoperfusion (Table 11-6)

TABLE 11-5. Gastrointestinal Decontamination

Therapy	Contraindications
Emesis - Syrup of Ipecac	
Dosage: • Less than 1 yr 10 ml • Young children 15 ml • Adolescents, adults 30 ml May repeat once	• Petroleum distillates • Common caustic agents • Stupor and/or coma • Rapid coma inducing drugs e.g., propoxyphene, TCA
Lavage	

• Large bore orogastric hose -
  28 F Ewald tube for young
  children, 36-40 suitable for
  adolescents
• Left recumbent
  Trendelenburg position to
  reduce the risk of aspiration
• Lavage with saline or 1/2 N
  saline until return is clear
	• Corrosive caustic agents
	• Controversial in petroleum
	  distillates ingestion
	• Stupor and/or coma unless
	  airway protected

Activated Charcoal	

Administer in all cases after
emesis
Dosage:
• Children   1 gm/kg
• Adults   50-100 gm
	• Corrosive agents: charcoal
	  interferes with GI endoscopy
	• Acetaminophen ingestion:
	  charcoal reduces absorption of
	  N-acetyl-cysteine

Cathartics	

• $MgSO_4$ 250 mg/kg/dose PO
  (max. dose 30 g) in 10-20%
  solution
• Sorbitol magnesium citrate
 	
Repeat above doses 2-4 hourly
until passage of charcoal stained
stools
	• Avoid $MgSO_4$ in renal failure

E. Antidotal therapy

Only a small proportion of poisoned patients are amenable to antidotal therapy (Table 11-7) and in only a few poisonings is antidotal therapy urgent, e.g., carbon monoxide, cyanide, organophosphate and narcotic intoxication.

TABLE 11-6. Removal of Common Intoxicants

Drug	Indicated for level (μg/dl)	Diuresis	Dialysis	HP[*]
Acetaminophen		No	No	No
Amphetamines		Yes	Yes	
Benzodiazepines		No	No	No
Ethanol		No	Yes	No
Ethylene glycol	>500	No	Yes	No
Ethchlorvynol	>150	No	Yes	Yes
Glutethimide	>40	No	Yes	
Isopropanol		No	Yes	No
Methanol	>500	No	Yes	No
Narcotics		No	No	No
Phencyclidine		Yes	No	
Phenobarbital	>100	Yes		
Salicylates	>800	Yes	Yes	Yes
	(lower if severe acidosis)			
Theophylline	>50 - 80	No	Yes	Yes
Tricyclic antidepressants		No	No	No

Adapted from Wanke LA, Bennett WM: Enhancement of elimination: diuresis, peritoneal dialysis, hemodialysis, and hemoperfusion. In Bayer MJ, Rumack BH, Wanke LA (eds): **Toxicologic Emergencies**, 1984. Reprinted by permission of Prentice-Hall, Inc., Englewood, NJ.
[*] HP - hemoperfusion

TABLE 11-7. Specific Intoxications and Their Antidotes

Poison	Antidote	Indications	Dose
Acetaminophen	N-Acetylcysteine (Mucomyst)	Serum acetaminophen level in "probable" hepatotoxic range (Figure 11-1)	140 mg/kg P.O. initial dose, then 70 mg/kg every 4 hr for 17 doses
Anticholinergics	Physostigmine	• Supraventricular tachycardia with hemodynamic compromise • Severe agitation	Adult: 1 mg IV Q 10 min (max 4 mg) Child: 0.5 mg IV Q 10 min to desired effect (max 2 mg)
Beta blockers	Glucagon	Bradycardia	Adult: 3 mg bolus, followed by 5 mg/hr infusion Child: 0.05 mg/kg bolus, followed by 0.07 mg/kg/hr infusion
	Isoproterenol, dopamine, epinephrine	Bradycardia	Infusion: titrate to effect
Carbon monoxide	Oxygen	Carbon monoxide levels > 5-10%	100% O_2. Consider hyperbaric oxygenation

Cyanide	Amyl nitrite, sodium nitrite; sodium thiosulfate	Symptomatic intoxication	**Adult:** Amyl nitrite inhalation pending administration of IV sodium nitrite 300 mg (3% solution) then sodium thiosulfate 12.5 gm (25% solution) **Child:** For children <25 kg sodium nitrite and sodium thiosulfate doses are dependent on the hemoglobin concentration, since an overdose can cause fatal methemoglobinemia - *
Ethylene glycol	Ethanol	• Osmolar gap and metabolic acidosis regardless of ethylene glycol level • Serum level > 20 mg/dl regardless of symptomatology	**Loading dose:** 7.6-10 ml/kg 10% ethanol in D_5W (loading dose) and maintenance infusion to achieve blood level of 100 mg. **Maintenance dose:** 1.4 ml/kg/hr. Infuse the sum of the loading dose and first hour's maintenance dose over the first hour
Iron salts	Desferoxamine	• Symptomatic patients • Serum iron > 350 μg/ml or serum iron > TIBC • Positive desferoxamine challenge test	Desferoxamine 15 mg/kg/hr or 40 mg/kg IM. Repeat every 4-8 hr until urine color is normal or iron level < 300 μg/dl.

Continued.

TABLE 11-7. (cont.).

Isoniazid	Pyridoxine (vit B₆)		For a known isoniazid dose, administer an equivalent amount of IV pyridoxine. If supplies are limited or the dose unknown, administer pyridoxine 5 gm. Cumulative dose is 20 gm in children and 40 gm in adults.
Methanol	Ethanol	• Metabolic acidosis and elevated osmolar gap regardless of symptoms	For dosage, see under **Ethylene glycol**
Methemoglobinemia producing agents (nitrites, nitrates, phenacetin, phenazopyridine)	Methylene blue	• Symptomatic poisoning • Methemoglobin level > 30-40%	1-2 mg/kg IV (0.1-0.2 ml/kg of a 1 % solution over 5-10 min) contraindicated in methemoglobinemia secondary to sodium nitrite administration for cyanide poisoning
Narcotics	Naloxone	Symptomatic intoxication	**Adult: 0.4 mg IV** **Child: 0.01 mg/kg IV** Repeat at 10 X dose if no response and findings are consistent with narcotic overdose

Organophosphate insecticides	Atropine	Cholinergic crisis	**Adult:** 2-5 mg IV **Child:** 0.05 mg/kg IV Repeat every 10-30 min to achieve adequate atropinization
	Pralidoxime (Protopam, 2-PAM)	Fasciculation and weakness	Only after atropine. **Adult:** 1 gm IV. **Child:** 25 mg/kg IV. Repeat after 1 hr if weakness and fasciculations persist
Phenothiazines	Diphenhydramine	Symptomatic intoxication- (oculogyric crisis)	0.5-1.0 mg/kg IV or IM (not to exceed 50 mg)

* Sodium Nitrate and Sodium Thiosulfate Doses for Cyanide Poisoning

Hemoglobin (g/100 ml)	Initial Dose 3% Na nitrite (ml/kg IV)	then	Initial Dose 25% Sodium Thiosulfate (ml/kg IV)
8	0.22		1.10
10	0.27		1.35
12	0.33		1.65
14	0.39		1.95

Adapted from: Henretig FM, Cupit AC, Temple AR: Toxicologic emergencies. In Ludwig S, Fleischer G (Eds): **Textbook of Pediatric Emergency Medicine.** Philadelphia, WB Saunders, 1983.

IV. ACETAMINOPHEN

Acetaminophen is present in many over-the-counter analgesic and antipyretic compounds. A dose of > 140 mg/kg is considered toxic in older children and adults; infants may be more resistant.

A. Clinical Manifestations

1. First 12-24 hours patients are either asymptomatic or develop nausea, anorexia, and vomiting.
2. Next 12-24 hours: There is resolution of earlier gastrointestinal symptoms.
3. After 72 hours liver injury may develop with marked elevation of transaminase, prolonged PT and PTT, and jaundice. Fulminant liver failure may occur but is not an inevitable occurrence.

B. Laboratory Tests

Measure serum acetaminophen levels.

C. Prediction of Toxicity

1. Toxicity likely with ingestion of > 140 mg/kg.
2. Rumack-Matthew nomogram (Figure 11-1) defines the risk of hepatic damage in terms of serum levels and duration from the time of ingestion. It is applicable only in **acute** intoxication.

D. Management

1. Gastrointestinal decontamination (Table 11-5).
2. Do not administer activated charcoal. It reduces the absorption of N-acetylcysteine.
3. Administer the antidote N-acetylcysteine up to 24 hours after ingestion if serum acetaminophen is either in the "possible" or "probable" hepatotoxic range (see nomogram, Figure 11-1).
4. If levels are unavailable, treat as if toxicity is possible. Stop therapy if levels are subsequently reported as non-toxic.
5. Dose N-acetylcysteine; 140 mg/kg as a 5% solution (diluted four-fold with juice or cola), followed by 70 mg/kg every 4 hr for 17 doses.

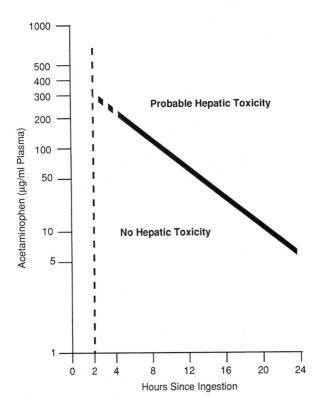

Figure 11-1. Rumack-Matthew nomogram for estimating likelihood of hepatic toxicity with acetaminophen intoxication using serum acetaminophen levels.
From: Rumack BH, Matthew H. Acetaminophen poisoning and toxicity. Pediatrics 55:871, 1975. Reproduced with permission of Pediatrics.

V. ANTICHOLINERGICS

Antihistamines, belladonna alkaloids, phenothiazines, butyrophenones, tricyclic antidepressants, gastrointestinal and genitourinary antispasmodics, antiparkinsonian drugs, over-the-counter cold remedies and sleep aids.

A. Clinical Manifestations

"**Hot** as a Hare, **Blind** as a Bat, **Dry** as a Bone, **Red** as a Beet, **Mad** as a Hatter".

1. Peripheral Anticholinergic Effects
    Tachycardia, hypertension, dry mucous membranes, flushed dry skin, fever, mydriasis, blurred vision, constipation and urinary retention.

2. Central Anticholinergic Effects
    Confusion, memory loss, agitation, movement disorder, hallucinations, convulsions, coma.

B. Laboratory Tests

Urine toxicology screen can detect anticholinergic compounds.

C. Management

1. Gastrointestinal decontamination (Table 11-5).

2. Administer the antidote physostigmine, a short acting, nonspecific cholinesterase inhibitor that will antagonize peripheral muscarinic blockade and central anticholinergic effects for:

    a. Severe hallucinations and agitation.

    b. Seizures unresponsive to conventional anticonvulsants.

    c. Coma (use as a diagnostic test).

    d. Supraventricular arrhythmias with hemodynamic compromise. Physostigmine is contraindicated in anticholinergic-induced ventricular arrhythmias. Lidocaine, phenytoin, or propranalol are preferred.)

VI. SALICYLATES

Aspirin or acetyl salicylic acid is available alone or in combination in many over-the-counter preparations. Other salicylate preparations include methylsalicylate (Oil of Wintergreen) and salicylic acid (a keratolytic).

A. Clinical Manifestations (Table 11-8)

Clinical manifestations are a reflection of a systemic illness caused by disturbed oxidative phosphorylation, alterations in carbohydrate, protein and lipid metabolism and direct stimulation of medullary respiratory centers.

TABLE 11-8. Clinical Manifestations of Salicylate Toxicity

Common	Uncommon
• Fever	• Respiratory depression
• Sweating	• Non-cardiogenic pulmonary edema
• Nausea	• Inappropriate ADH release syndrome
• Vomiting	• Hemolysis
• Coagulopathy, bleeding	• Renal failure
• Dehydration	• Hepatotoxicity
• Hyperpnea	• Cerebral edema
• Tinnitus	
• Seizures	
• Coma	

B. Laboratory Findings in Salicylism (Table 11-9)

C. Prediction of toxicity

1. Ingested dose can predict the severity of an acute intoxication (Table 11-10).

TABLE 11-9. Laboratory Findings in Salicylate Toxicity

- Metabolic acidosis
- Respiratory alkalosis
- Mixed respiratory alkalosis and metabolic acidosis
- Hyperglycemia, hypoglycemia
- Hyponatremia, hypernatremia
- Hypokalemia
- Hypocalcemia
- Prolonged prothrombin time
- Urine ketones positive
- Urine ferric chloride test or Phenistix test positive

TABLE 11-10. Prediction of Acute Salicylate Toxicity

Ingested Dose (mg/kg)	Potential Severity of Toxicity
• < 150	• Toxicity not expected
• 150-300	• Mild to moderate
• 300-500	• Severe
• > 500	• Potentially lethal

From Temple AR: Acute and chronic effects of aspirin toxicity and their treatment. Arch Intern Med. 141:366, 1981. Copyright, 1981, American Medical Association.

2. Serum salicylate level can predict severity of intoxication. (In acute overdose, measure serum salicylate level 6 hours after ingestion.)
   a. Done nomogram (Figure 11-2) defines the expected severity of intoxication in terms of serum salicylate levels at various intervals following ingestion.

    b.   Only predictive in single ingestion, acute intoxication.

    c.   Poor correlation between serum salicylate levels and the severity of chronic intoxication. May have moderately severe chronic salicylate toxicity with therapeutic serum salicylate level.

  3.   Clinical manifestations reflect severity of both acute and chronic salicylate intoxication. (Table 11-11).

TABLE 11-11. Manifestations of Severity of Aspirin Intoxication

Severity Category	Symptoms
• Asymptomatic	• None
• Mild	• Mild-moderate hyperpnea, sometimes with lethargy
• Moderate	• Severe hyperpnea, prominent neurologic disturbances (marked lethargy and/or excitability), but no coma or convulsions
• Severe	• Severe hyperpnea, coma, or semicoma, sometimes with convulsions

From Temple AR: Acute and chronic effects of aspirin toxicity and their treatment. Arch Intern Med. 141:366, 1981. Copyright 1981, American Medical Association.

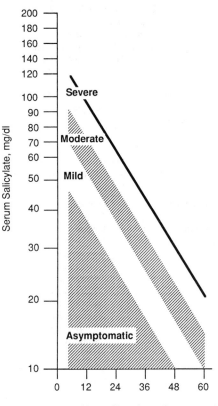

Hours Since Ingestion

Figure 11-2. The Done nomogram for estimating the severity of salicylate poisoning using serum salicylate levels.
From: Temple AR: Acute and chronic effects of aspirin toxicity and their treatment. Arch Intern Med 141:366, 1981. Copyright 1981, American Medical Association.

D. **Management**

1. GI decontamination (Table 11-5)
2. General supportive care.
    a. Correct dehydration by administering 10-20 ml/kg of 0.45 NS + 35-75 mEq HCO_3/L. For moderate or severe toxicity: forced alkaline diuresis using the above solution with 40-60 mEq KCl/L added after urine output has been established. The goal is to achieve a urine output >2 ml/kg/hour and urine pH >7.5. Forced diuresis is contraindicated in the presence of cerebral edema, pulmonary edema and renal failure.
    b. Treat acidosis (IV $NaHCO_3$).
    c. Monitor electrolytes, glucose, calcium and replace if necessary.
    d. Vitamin K for hemorrhagic diathesis.
    e. Decrease fever with external cooling.
    f. Dialysis

       Hemodialysis is more efficient than peritoneal dialysis. Indications for dialysis include severe intoxication (Done nomogram), severe acidosis unresponsive to $NaHCO_3$, renal failure, pulmonary edema and severe CNS manifestations.

VII. IRON

The severity of iron intoxication is directly related to the amount of elemental iron ingested. The iron content of ferrous gluconate, sulphate and fumarate is 12, 20 and 33% respectively.

A. **Clinical Manifestations**

1. Phase 1

   First 6 hours. Nausea, vomiting, diarrhea, abdominal pain, hematemesis, melena.

2. Phase 2
   6 to 12 hours. Temporary recovery and deceptive quiescence.
3. Phase 3
   Recrudescence of gastrointestinal manifestations with jaundice, metabolic acidosis, shock, hyperglycemia, hemorrhagic diathesis, central nervous system depression progressing to coma and death.
4. Phase 4
   Gastrointestinal scarring with either pyloric, gastric or intestinal stenosis at 4-6 weeks.

B. Laboratory Tests

1. Measure serum iron and total iron binding capacity (TIBC) 2-4 hours after ingestion. After 6 hours, iron has been rapidly cleared from serum by the liver. Thus, low iron levels can be measured in a potentially lethally intoxicated patient.
2. Ancillary laboratory tests with moderate or severe ingestion should include complete blood count, glucose, blood gas, BUN, electrolytes, PT, PTT, liver enzymes (AST and ALT).
3. X-ray the abdomen after emesis or lavage to detect residual pill fragments.

C. Prediction of Toxicity
1. Dose of elemental Fe ingested (Table 11-12).

TABLE 11-12. Ingested Iron Load and Toxicity

Potential Severity	Amount Fe Ingested
• Insignificant	• < 20 mg/kg
• Moderate	• 20-60 mg/kg
• Potentially lethal	• > 200 mg/kg

---

2. Serum iron level (Table 11-13)
    The normal serum iron level range is 50-100
    μg/dl. Serum levels in excess of TIBC is diag-
    nostic of iron intoxication (normal TIBC 300-400
    μg/dl).

TABLE 11-13. Serum Iron Level and Toxicity

Iron level (μg/dl)	Potential Severity
• < 100	• Insignificant
• 100-300	• Minimal
• 300-350	• Moderate
• 500-1000	• Severe
• > 1000	• Potentially lethal

From: Henretig FM, Temple AR: Acute iron poisoning. Emerg
Med Clin North Am 2:121, 1984.

---

3. Desferoxamine challenge test
    Desferoxamine test may be helpful in estimating
    severity and need for therapy when serum iron
    determinations are not readily available in moder-
    ately symptomatic patients.

    Administer deferoxamine 40 mg/kg IM or 15
    mg/kg IV for 1 hour. The appearance of vin rosé
    colored urine indicates the presence of free iron in
    excess of the iron binding capacity and the need
    for continued chelation therapy. However, urine
    does not always change color in spite of serum
    iron level that exceeds TIBC.

D. Management

1. Gastrointestinal decontamination (Table 11-5)
    When post-emesis abdominal x-ray reveals radio-opaque material, perform gastric lavage. The use of either $NaHCO_3$ or desferoxamine containing lavage solutions is controversial.

2. Chelation therapy indications
    a. Symptomatic patient (gastrointestinal symptoms together with lethargy, tachypnea, hypoperfusion and tachycardia).
    b. Serum iron level > 350 μg/dl or serum iron $>$ TIBC (Table 11-13).
    c. Positive desferoxamine challenge test.

3. Chelation therapy dose
    a. Desferoxamine 15 mg/kg/hr IV. Hypotension can develop with more rapid administration. May give 40 mg/kg IM if less severely intoxicated.
    b. Continue until the urine is no longer vin rosé in color (if it becomes discolored with the initial dose) or until serum iron level $<$ 300 μg/dl.

VIII. ALCOHOLS: ETHANOL, METHANOL, ISOPROPANOL AND ETHYLENE GLYCOL

Ethanol is the most commonly used mood altering drug. In children, ingestion of the other three alcohols is generally accidental, although occasionally they are ingested as ethanol substitutes.

A.   Clinical Manifestations (Table 11-14)

TABLE 11-14.   Clinical Manifestations of Alcohol Intoxication

---

Ethanol	CNS depression, slurred speech, muscular incoordination, coma, respiratory depression. Hypoglycemia in children. Alcohol breath odor.
Methanol	Initial phase of mild inebriation followed by asymptomatic 6-24 hours. Subsequent headaches, vomiting, CNS depression, visual disturbances with retinal edema. Metabolic acidosis. Formaldehyde odor on breath.
Isopropanol	Clinical features resemble ethanol with predominant CNS depression including confusion, nystagmus, and coma. Gastrointestinal symptoms with abdominal pain, vomiting, and hematemesis. Acetone breath odor
Ethylene glycol	Phase 1: CNS depression, confusion, nausea and vomiting. No breath odor. Phase 2: Cardio-respiratory failure Phase 3: Renal failure.

B.   Laboratory Tests

Laboratory test results in the differential diagnosis of intoxication by the alcohols are outlined in Table 11-15.

1.   Measure blood levels of the alcohols. (Use gas chromatography since enzymatic method utilizing alcohol dehydrogenase will not distinguish between these alcohols. This is important since early antidotal therapy is crucial with ethylene glycol and methanol intoxication).

2. Measure anion gap, osmolar gap (Table 11-4), arterial blood gas, glucose, electrolytes, and calcium.
3. Urinalysis for ketones and oxalate crystals.

TABLE 11-15. Laboratory Findings in Patients Intoxicated with the Alcohols

	Ethanol	Methanol	Isopropyl alcohol	Ethylene glycol
Osmolar gap	Present	Present	Present	Present
Metabolic acidosis (increased anion gap)	Mild-moderate (adults with chronic abuse)	Severe	None-mild	Severe
Ketosis	Alcoholic keto-acidosis (adult chronic abuse)	None	Marked	None
Other laboratory findings	↓ Glucose	↑ amy-lase, ↓ Ca	↓ Glucose	↑ BUN, ↑ creati-nine, ↓ Na

C. Management

1. Gastrointestinal contamination (Table 11-5).
2. Treat metabolic acidosis with $NaHCO_3$ (methanol, ethylene glycol poisoning).

3. Administer ethanol for methanol and ethylene glycol intoxication to competitively inhibit alcohol dehydrogenase and reduce the production of toxic metabolites.

Loading dose (to achieve serum level of 100 mg/dl) 7.6-10 ml/kg of 10% ethanol in D_5W, then maintenance dose of 1.4 ml/kg/hour.

4. Dialysis (hemodialysis)

Indications include methanol and ethylene glycol serum levels > 50 mg/dl, severe metabolic acidosis resistant to $NaHCO_3$ therapy, and renal failure in ethylene glycol poisoning.

IX. ORGANOPHOSPHATE AND CARBAMATE INSECTICIDES

These are potent acetylcholinesterase inhibitors that are rapidly absorbed from the gastrointestinal tract and skin.

A. Clinical Manifestations (Table 11-16)

B. Laboratory Tests

1. Red blood cell cholinesterase and serum pseudo-cholinesterase.
2. Chest x-ray, arterial blood gas
3. ECG
4. Toxicological examination of urine for metabolic byproducts of organophosphates e.g., p-nitrophenol.

TABLE 11-16. Organophosphate and Carbamate Poisoning

Anatomic Site	Manifestation
Central nervous system effects	Headache, lethargy, restlessness, dizziness, confusion, coma, seizures, respiratory depression, convulsions
Nicotinic effects	
Skeletal muscle	Cramps, fasciculations, weakness, paralysis
Sympathetic ganglia	Tachycardia, hypertension, arrhythmias, pallor, mydriasis
Muscarinic effects	
Cardiac	Bradycardia, hypotension, heart block, arrhythmias
Respiratory	Bronchorrhea, wheezing, respiratory distress
Gastrointestinal	Cramps, vomiting, nausea, diarrhea, tenesmus, abdominal pain
Salivary glands	Excess salivation
Sweat glands	Sweating
Eyes	Miosis, lacrimation, blurred vision
Bladder	Incontinence
Miscellaneous	Garlic odor, fever

From Haddad LM: The organophosphate insecticides. In Haddad LM, Winchester JF (eds). Clinical Management of Poisoning and Drug Overdose. Philadelphia, WB Saunders, 1983.

C. Management

1. Skin decontamination.
2. Gastrointestinal decontamination (Table 11-5).
3. Administer antidotes atropine and pralidoxime.

   a. Atropine

   Atropine blocks the effects of acetylcholine in the CNS and muscarinic receptors but has no effect on the neuromuscular junction (nicotinic receptor).

   Dose: Child, 0.05 mg/kg IV. Adult, 2-5 mg IV q 5 min until therapeutic response (decreased oral and bronchial secretions). Once atropinization is achieved, repeat q 30 min. Enormous doses exceeding 0.5 mg/kg per 24 hours may be needed.

   b. Pralidoxime

   Pralidoxime regenerates active cholinesterase by displacing inhibitor from enzyme-inhibitor complex. Indications for use are muscle weakness, paralysis, fasciculations. Only administer after atropinization.

   Dose: 25 mg/kg IV (child); 1-2 gm IV (adult). Repeat q 1 hour if fasciculations and weakness persist.

D. Management - Carbamate Poisoning

The pathophysiology of carbamate poisoning differs from organophosphate poisoning in two important respects. First, the carbamates only temporarily inactivate cholinesterase. Second, they penetrate the CNS only poorly. The clinical manifestations thus resemble those of organophosphate poisoning but are of short duration and lack the signs and symptoms of CNS involvement. The treatment of carbamate intoxication is only atropine administration. Pralidoxime need not be administered.

X.   THEOPHYLLINE

Theophylline-containing compounds are the most frequently prescribed pharmaceuticals for the treatment of asthma. Widespread availability and a narrow therapeutic index make theophylline toxicity a common problem.

A.   Clinical Manifestations
1. Gastrointestinal: nausea, vomiting, abdominal pain.
2. Cardiac: supraventricular and ventricular arrhythmias (secondary to a hyperadrenergic state).
3. Neurological - agitation, hyperpnea, tremors, lethargy, coma, seizures.
4. Metabolic abnormalities - hypokalemia, hyperglycemia, hypophosphatemia, metabolic acidosis.

B.   Laboratory Tests
Measure theophylline level, electrolytes, glucose, blood gases.

C.   Prediction of Toxicity
Serum theophylline does not necessarily reflect the severity of toxicity. High serum levels produced by acute intoxication are generally better tolerated than the same levels achieved by chronic administration.

D.   Management
1. Gastrointestinal decontamination (Table 11-5)
2. Repeat doses of activated charcoal q 2 hours. This reduces elimination half life ("intestinal dialysis").
3. Charcoal hemoperfusion. Indications are unclear but include:
   a. seizures, arrhythmias, hypotension unresponsive to conventional medical therapy,
   b. serum levels greater than 80-100 μg/ml.

4. Seizures - administer diazepam 0.1-0.2 mg/kg IV.
5. Arrhythmias (*Chapter 7*)
    a. Supraventricular - specific treatment usually not indicated.
    b. Ventricular - Administer lidocaine 1 mg/kg IV.

XI. TRICYCLIC ANTIDEPRESSANTS (TCA)

TCA consist of tertiary (amitriptyline, imipramine, doxepin) and secondary (nortriptyline, desipramine, and protriptyline) amines. Tetracyclics (maprotiline and amoxapine) resemble the TCA toxicologically.

A. Mechanisms of Toxicity
1. Central and peripheral anticholinergic actions.
2. Decreased reuptake of norepinephrine in adrenergic nerve endings enhances catecholamine action in the central nervous system and peripheral nerve tissues.
3. "Quinidine like" myocardial depressant effect.

B. Clinical Manifestations (Table 11-17)

C. Laboratory Tests
TCA can be detected in blood and urine but serum levels have no particular implications for therapy.

D. Prediction of Toxicity
1. Dose ingested
   10-20 mg/kg of most tricyclics - moderate, severe toxicity.
2. Prolonged QRS interval (reflection of "quinidine like" myocardial depressant effect) > 100 msec
   A prolonged QRS interval correlates with the severity of TCA intoxication and with a serum level of > 1000 ng/ml. Use limb-lead QRS duration since the chest lead QRS interval duration is

tion since the chest lead QRS interval duration is 0.01-0.02 sec longer than the limb lead QRS complexes.

TABLE 11-17.   Manifestations of Tricyclic Antidepressant Intoxication

---

SITE OF ACTION	SIGN OR SYMPTOM
• CNS effects	Drowsiness, lethargy, delirium, agitation, hallucinations, respiratory depression, coma, movement disorders (twitching, myoclonic jerks, pyramidal tract signs, choreoathetosis)
• Peripheral anticholinergic effects	Dry mucous membranes, flushed warm skin without sweating, mydriasis, blurred vision, urinary retention, ileus
• Cardiovascular effects (due to 3 pharmacological effects) 1. blockage of norepinephrine reuptake 2. anticholinergic effects 3. "quinidine like" myocardial depressant effects	Hypotension, Arrhythmias • 2nd & 3rd degree block; right bundle branch block; nonspecific intraventricular delay pattern • tachyarrhythmias: supraventricular and ventricular tachycardias, ventricular fibrillation, premature ventricular beats

---

E.   Management

1.   Gastrointestinal decontamination (Table 11-5).
2.   Repeat charcoal administration q 4 hours to interrupt the enterohepatic circulation of TCA.

Physostigmine (Table 11-7) reverses CNS and peripheral anticholinergic symptoms but is usually unnecessary. Seizures are best treated with diazepam 0.1-0.2 mg/kg IV. Physostigmine may be used for resistant seizures. Coma per se is not an indication for physostigmine.

4. Treatment of arrhythmias and hypotension (Table 11-20)

TABLE 11-18. **Treatment of Cardiovascular Complications of Tricyclic Antidepressant Intoxication**

Hypotension	• Fluid administration. • Vasoactive drugs. Use direct-acting alpha agents, e.g., neosynephrine, norepinephrine rather than catecholamine precursor drugs e.g., dopamine.
Ventricular arrhythmias	• Alkalinization (pH 7.45-7.55) with NaHCO$_3$, and/or hyperventilation. • If alkalinization fails, administer lidocaine or phenytoin as second line therapy. • Avoid quinidine, procainamide, and disopyramide. • Propranolol can be used for supraventricular tachycardia. • Physostigmine is not effective in treating TCA induced arrhythmias.
Heart block (2nd/ 3rd degree)	• Alkalinization. • Beta agonist chronotropes (e.g., epinephrine). • Pacing. • Physostigmine and phenytoin contraindicated.

XII. OPIOIDS

A. Clinical Manifestations of Toxicity
Respiratory depression, miosis, and depressed consciousness characterize opioid intoxication (Table 11-19).

TABLE 11-19. Clinical Manifestations of Opioid Toxicity

Clinical Manifestations	Comments
Central Nervous System	
• Coma	• All opioids
• Seizures	• Particularly propoxyphene
• Miosis	• Meperidine less consistently Lomotil (diphenoxylate and atropine), may produce mydriasis
Cardiovascular	
• Hypotension	• All opioids. Aggravated by hypoxia.
• Arrhythmias	• Uncommon
	• Atrial fibrillation particularly with heroin overdose
	• Prolonged QRS particularly with propoxyphene overdose
Pulmonary	
• Respiratory depression	• All opioids
• Pulmonary edema	• Noncardiogenic etiology
Miscellaneous	• Ileus, nausea

B. Laboratory Tests

1. Toxicology screen (urine for qualitative detection of opioids).
2. Blood gas determination, if indicated.

C. Treatment

1. Resuscitation and stabilization.
2. GI decontamination (Table 11-5).
3. Antidotal therapy - naloxone (See *Chapter 10*)
    a. Dose 0.01 mg/kg. Note: Supplied as 0.02 mg/ml for neonatal use and 0.4 mg/ml for all others. If ineffective, give up to 10 times the starting dose.
    b. Since duration of action of most narcotics is longer than that of naloxone, administer additional doses of naloxone or titrate to effect with a continuous infusion (1-5 μg/kg/min).

XIII. HYDROCARBONS

Accidentally ingested hydrocarbons include the petroleum distillates (kerosene, lighter fluid, seal oil, gasoline, furniture oil), and pine oil distillates (turpentine).

The toxicity of these agents is due primarily to pulmonary aspiration and not to systemic absorption. The risk of aspiration is higher with low viscosity, highly volatile compounds (gasoline, kerosene and mineral seal oil) than with low viscosity oils (lubricating oil, petrolatum, paraffin). Toxic additives that include heavy metals, pesticides, toluene, and camphor produce additional toxicity.

A. Clinical Manifestations (Table 11-20)

TABLE 11-20. Clinical Manifestations of Hydrocarbon Toxicity

Clinical Manifestations	Comments
Respiratory	
• Cough, respiratory distress, dyspnea, cyanosis, hemoptysis, wheezes, rales, fever (chest x-ray reveals aspiration pneumonia)	• Due to aspiration. Usually present within 6 hours if aspiration has occurred.
CNS	
• CNS depression, somnolence	• Uncommon. Probably due to hypoxia since systemic absorption of hydrocarbons is small. May be due to toxicity of additives.
Gastrointestinal	
• Nausea, vomiting, abdominal pain, diarrhea	
Hematological	
• Hemolysis, hemoglobinemia	• Occurs with gasoline ingestion (from red cell membrane damage)

B. Laboratory Findings

1. Chest x-ray
2. CBC and blood gases, if clinically indicated. Tests to identify poisoning from toxic additives to petroleum distillates e.g., aniline or nitrobenzene (methemoglobin), organophosphates and heavy metals.

C. Treatment

1. Resuscitation and stabilization.
2. GI decontamination (Table 11-5). Indications for emesis or lavage are controversial and not universally accepted. Emesis or lavage is not indicated for ingestion of commonly ingested hydrocarbons that do not contain toxic additives. Induce emesis or lavage with the ingestion of toxic additives e.g., camphor, pesticides, aniline, toluene, nitrobenzene, chlorinated hydrocarbons, xylene, benzene.

Chapter 12
MENINGITIS AND SEPSIS

I. OVERVIEW

A. Bacterial Meningitis
Bacterial meningitis in children carries a high morbidity (30-50%) and mortality (5-10%), despite continued advances in antibiotic and adjunctive therapy.

B. Outcome
The outcome from severe sepsis varies according to the infecting organism, the child's age, and state of immune competence.

C. Approach
An organized initial approach is needed for evaluation and treatment of life-threatening sepsis or meningitis in infants and children (Figure 12-1).
1. Attention first to stabilization of airway, breathing, circulation (ABC's).
2. Obtain enough information (based on brief history and limited physical exam) to make presumptive diagnosis (Table 12-1) and choose appropriate antibiotics (Table 12-2).

TABLE 12-1. Some Findings Suggestive of Infection

- Fever
- Rash
- Sudden cardiovascular collapse
- Signs of meningeal or peritoneal irritation
- Altered mental status
- Respiratory abnormalities
- Lymphadenopathy
- Joint swelling

Approach to Life-Threatening Infections

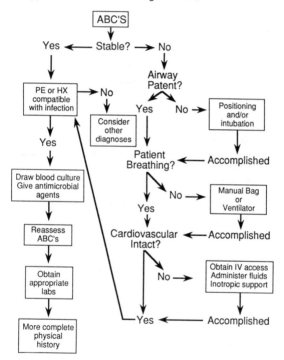

Figure 12-1. Approach to life-threatening infections.

TABLE 12-2. Appropriate Initial Antibiotics

AGE	ANTIBIOTIC	STARTING DOSE (mg/kg/dose)
Newborn	AMPICILLIN and	<7 days: 25-50 q12h >7 days: 30-70 q8h
	either GENTAMICIN	<7 days (term): 2.5 q12h >7 days (term): 2.5 q8h
	or CEFOTAXIME	<7 days: 25-50 q12h >7 days: 25-50 q8h
1-3 mos	AMPICILLIN and	50-100 q6h
either	CEFOTAXIME or	12.5-45 q6h
	CEFTRIAXONE or	1st DOSE: 75, then 50 q12h
	AMIKACIN or GENTAMICIN	5 q8h 1.7-2.5 q8h
≥ 3 mos	either AMPICILLIN and CHLORAMPHENICOL	50-100 q6h 25 q6h
	or CEFTRIAXONE alone	see above (max=2g/day)
	or CEFOTAXIME alone	see above (max=12g/day)

3. Obtain additional history (Table 12-3) and evaluate laboratory data. Decide whether to perform a lumbar puncture in comatose child. Differential diagnosis of coma includes trauma, mass lesions, and toxins.

TABLE 12-3. Important Historical Information

- Recent travel
- Menses history (tampon use)
- Animal or insect bites
- Immunization status
- Known exposures
- Risk group for HIV, other immunodeficiency states

II. INFECTION IN THE NEONATE (Table 12-4)

TABLE 12-4. Neonatal Sepsis and Meningitis: Bacterial Agents

SEPSIS	MENINGITIS
Frequent Causes	
Escherichia coli	*Escherichia coli*
Group B Streptococcus	Group B Streptococcus
Klebsiella-Enterobacter-Citrobacter	
Occasional Causes	
Staphylococcus aureus	*Streptococcus pneumoniae*
Staphylococcus epidermidis	Staphylococcus species
Alpha-hemolytic Streptococcus	*Haemophilus influenzae*, type b
Anaerobic Gram negative	Proteus, Pseudomonas
	Listeria monocytogenes
	Klebsiella, Aerobacter
	Salmonella species
Rare Causes	
Group D Streptococcus	Streptococcus species
Anaerobic Streptococci	*Neisseria meningitidis, N. gonorrhoeae*
Group A Streptococcus	Citrobacter, Enterobacter
	Anaerobic Gram negative
	Flavobacterium meningosepticum

A. *Group B Streptococcus* (GBS)

1. Epidemiology
   Epidemiologic studies show a bimodal distribution of GBS sepsis (Table 12-5). The majority (75%) present in first week of life, usually in first 48 hours. Late onset is after first week, through third month of life.

TABLE 12-5. Clinical Characteristics of Group B Strep

	Early onset	Late onset
Peak age at onset	First 48 hrs	3-4 weeks
Incidence per 1000 live births	3.5 - 4	0.5 - 1.5
Presentation	Fulminant acute onset Apnea Respiratory distress Cardiovascular collapse Meningitis in 30 %	Less fulminant Meningitis in 75% May have evidence of focal points: - septic arthritis - osteomyelitis
Risk factors	Low birth weight (<2500 g) Low Apgar score Twin gestation Maternal fever Ruptured membranes >12 hrs Premature labor (<35 weeks) Maternal colonization	No specific risk factors
Mortality	50%	10 - 20%

2.   Treatment of GBS

   a.   Penicillin alone is not adequate due to increasing number of strains tolerant to the drug. Currently suggested regimens are penicillin and gentamicin, or cefotaxime or ceftriaxone (see Table 12-2).

   b.   Adjunctive measures are used in some centers. None have been of widely proven benefit.
      (1)   granulocyte transfusions
      (2)   double volume exchange with fresh whole blood
      (3)   intravenous immunoglobulins (IVIG)

B. *Listeria monocytogenes*

1.   Uncommon but important cause of disease in neonates and pregnant women.

2.   Bimodal presentation like GBS, but may also result in <u>fetal</u> death, malformation, or induction of premature labor. Early onset disease has very high mortality (70%). Late onset has a better prognosis.

3.   Treatment

   Ampicillin is drug of choice. During the first 10-14 days of therapy combine ampicillin with gentamicin. Continue therapy with another 7 days of ampicillin alone.

C. *Herpes Simplex* Virus (HSV)

1.   May be indistinguishable from bacterial sepsis.
2.   Only 20-30% have mucosal or skin lesions.

3. 50% of babies develop meningoencephalitis, but many have normal cerebrospinal fluid (CSF) findings early on.
4. Suspect (HSV) in any neonate who fails to respond rapidly to antibiotics.
5. Treatment: (often started empirically) acyclovir - 30 mg/kg/day in three divided doses for 10-14 days.

III. OLDER INFANT AND CHILD

A different set of organisms is responsible for serious infections in the older child (Table 12-6).

TABLE 12-6. Causative Organisms in Sepsis and Meningitis of the Older Infant and Child

---

SEPSIS	MENINGITIS
Frequent Causes	
S. pneumoniae	H. influenzae, type b
H. influenzae, type b	S. pneumoniae
N. meningitidis	N. meningitidis
Less Frequent Causes	
S. aureus	Staph. species
S. pyogenes	Streptococcus species
Salmonella species	E. coli
Microaerophilic streptococcus	P. aeruginosa
	Klebsiella species
	Proteus species

A. N. meningitidis

1. May be rapidly fatal.
2. Incidence - highest in first year, drops to constant level by 10 years.

3. Presents as primarily sepsis or meningitis. Signs and symptoms vary (Table 12-7).
4. Laboratory data vary with severity (Table 12-8).

TABLE 12-7. Signs and Incidence of *N. meningitidis* Infection

---

- High fever (>40°C in 60%)
- Rash (macular, petechial or purpuric) (>60%)
- Meningeal signs (80%)
- Hypotension
- Tachycardia
- Tachypnea

TABLE 12-8.   Harbingers of Poor Prognosis in Meningococcal Disease

---

- Low white blood count
- Low platelet count
- Absence of meningitis
- Rapid onset of purpura

---

5. Prognosis
    Death occurs in 20% of patients. Majority of deaths take place in first 72 hours. Fulminant disease is associated with bilateral adrenal hemorrhage (Waterhouse-Friderichsen syndrome) and shock, not responsive to steroids (85% mortality).

6. Treatment
    a. Penicillin is drug of choice once diagnosis established. Broad spectrum coverage is necessary initially (penicillin and chloramphenicol or ceftriaxone) to cover

other organisms associated with petechiae (Table 12-9).

TABLE 12-9. Infectious Agents Associated with Petechiae

N. meningitidis	Mycoplasma
H. influenzae type b	*Epstein-Barr* virus
N. gonorrhoeae	Cytomegalovirus
S. pneumoniae	Colorado tick fever
S. pyogenes	Arboviruses
Enteroviruses	Rat-bite fever
Rubella	*Y. pestis*
Rickettsiae	

---

    b.   Supportive care may include:
       (1)   Volume expansion
       (2)   Inotropic support with dopamine and dobutamine
       (3)   Afterload reduction with nitroprusside
       (4)   Respiratory support including positive end expiratory pressure (PEEP)
       (5)   Pulse oximetry
       (6)   Invasive hemodynamic monitoring
       (7)   Intracranial pressure (ICP) monitoring

7.   Complications of infection
    a.   Arthritis
    b.   Deafness
    c.   Gastroenteritis
    d.   Pneumonia
    e.   Myocarditis-pericarditis-tamponade
    f.   Soft-tissue necrosis
    g.   Coagulopathy

8. Rifampin prophylaxis
    a. Indication
       All household, nursery school and day care contacts.
    b. Dose
       10 mg/kg/dose (maximum 600 mg) twice daily for 2 days.

B. *Haemophilus influenzae* type b

1. Most common cause of bacterial meningitis in children less than 5 years of age.
2. Also causes a host of other infections (Table 12-10).

TABLE 12-10. Diseases Caused by *H. influenzae* type b

Disease	Percent
Meningitis	51.0
Epiglottitis	17.4
Pneumonia	14.6
Arthritis	7.6
Cellulitis	6.0
Bacteremia	1.9
Osteomyelitis	1.6

3. Fulminant course is possible - similar to meningococcemia. May require supportive care as in III.A.6.b. (page 249).

4. Antibiotic therapy
    a. High percentage of organisms are beta-lactamase-producing and therefore inactivate penicillins.
    b. Drugs of choice
       (1) Third-generation cephalosporin (ceftriaxone or cefotaxime)

(2) Chloramphenicol (used less frequently now than in past)

5. Rifampin prophylaxis
    a. All household contacts in which at least one member is less than 48 months of age (including the index case).
    b. Dose - 20 mg/kg/dose, once daily for 4 days (maximum of 600 mg/dose).

6. Immunization not helpful in contacts.

IV. CRITICAL AND CONTROVERSIAL ISSUES

A. Lumbar Puncture (LP)
1. Best opportunity to make an etiologic diagnosis in infant or child with suspected meningitis.
2. May be dangerous in critically ill child (Table 12-11).
3. Stabilization of child (ABC's) should occur prior to LP.
4. Antibiotic therapy should not be delayed if LP is put off. Blood culture may yield organism. Urine for latex agglutination is also helpful.

TABLE 12-11. Relative Contraindications to Performance of an LP

- Airway incompetence
- Respiratory failure (actual or impending)
- Hemodynamic instability (shock)
- Bleeding diathesis (disseminated intravascular coagulopathy or severe thrombocytopenia)
- Possible increased intracranial pressure - coma, abnormal pupils, posturing, seizures

---

B. Intracranial Pressure Monitoring

1. Cerebral edema may occur in acute stages of meningitis which leads to cerebral ischemia or herniation.
2. Treat signs of increased ICP with intubation and hyperventilation.
3. CT scan is necessary to rule out mass lesions such as abscess or effusion.
4. ICP monitoring may be used to guide therapy in the absence of surgically amenable lesion, although there is no evidence to support improved outcome with aggressive ICP therapy.

C. Intravenous Immunoglobulins (IVIG)
Little documented efficacy except possibly in early GBS sepsis.

D. Steroids
1. Early studies in 1960's showed no effect of methylprednisolone 40 mg every 6 hours.
2. Studies of dexamethasone 0.15 mg/kg/dose every 6 hours with cefuroxime or ceftriaxone in patients with meningitis gave the following results (Lebel, N. Engl. J. Med. 319:964, 1988)
   a. Lower incidence of hearing loss in patients who received dexamethasone, significant only for patients with *Haemophilus influenzae* type b meningitis.
   b. The control rate of hearing loss in patients treated with cefuroxime alone was higher than national average.
   c. Increased risk of gastro-intestinal bleeding in the steroid treated group.
   d. Rate of CSF sterilization unchanged.

Chapter 13
ENVIRONMENTAL INJURIES

I. HYPOTHERMIA OVERVIEW

A. Definition
Hypothermia exists in the presence of an internal core temperature of 35°C (95°F) or less. Core temperature reflects the average temperature of the brain, heart, lungs, and viscera.

B. Etiology
The causes of hypothermia fall into 3 broad categories (Table 13-1) including:
1. Accidental: These are more frequently associated with the young infant, the elderly, the inebriated, and following immersion accidents.
2. Associated with chronic medical illnesses.
3. Secondary to acute illness: the most common acute cause in children is shock.

TABLE 13-1. Etiology of Hypothermia

Accidental:	Chronic illness:	Acute illness
- old age	- myxedema	- shock
- infancy	- pituitary insufficiency	- intoxication
- immersion	- Addison's disease	- sepsis
- alcohol	- pancreatitis	- hypoglycemia
intoxication	- cerebrovascular disease	- acute respiratory
	- Wernicke's encephalopathy	failure
	- myocardial infarction	- congestive heart
	- cirrhosis	failure

C. Physiology of Temperature Control

Normothermia (36°-37.5°C) depends on the balance between heat loss versus heat production and conservation.

1. Mechanisms of heat loss
   Heat loss occurs via the four mechanisms of:

   a. Radiation (transfer of heat to the surrounding environment by nonparticulate means, e.g., uncovered infant in a room with cold walls);
   b. Conduction (transfer of heat by direct contact with a stationary medium, e.g., cold water drowning);
   c. Convection (transfer of heat to moving air which is temporarily in contact with the body surface, e.g., increased heat loss during high winds in cold environment);
   d. Evaporation (heat lost during conversion of a liquid into a vapor, e.g., wet baby after birth).

2. Mechanisms of heat production/conservation
   Temperature control is integrated via the anterior hypothalamus such that cooling of the hypothalamus results in vasoconstriction (heat conservation) and shivering (heat production). Increased muscle tone and increased metabolic rate from sympathetic stimulation increase heat production by about four times the normal rate.

3. Infant vulnerability to hypothermia
   Infants are very prone to hypothermia because of increased risks of heat loss and inability to produce heat through shivering.

  a. Heat loss in infants is more likely because of minimal subcutaneous tissue, large surface area relative to weight, large head relative to body size.

  b. The newborn and infant (<3 mo.) are unable to shiver and depend on metabolism of brown fat for thermogenesis. Brown fat is highly vascular, rich in mitochondria, and located next to major vessels in the neck, chest, and abdomen. Hypothermia results in the release of norepinephrine which initiates the metabolism of brown fat to produce heat.

D. Physiologic Consequences of Hypothermia

Each organ system evolves through a characteristic sequence of changes as hypothermia becomes more prolonged and severe.

  1. Cardiovascular consequences
      Sympathetic stimulation results in tachycardia, increased cardiac output and mean arterial pressure during the early phases of mild hypothermia. Peripheral vasoconstriction redirects blood flow from extremities to the central circulation. Severe hypothermia may produce bradycardia, prolonged QT interval, atrial fibrillation, and ultimately ventricular tachycardia. Peripheral edema results from cell membrane Na^+/K^+ pump dysfunction such that Na^+ and water escape into the interstitial space.

  2. Respiratory consequences
      Tachypnea is found with mild hypothermia, but respiratory rate and tidal volume fall during severe hypothermia. Bronchiolar edema and decreased mucociliary function may lead to pulmonary infection. The oxyhemoglobin dissociation curve is

shifted to the left resulting in decreased unloading of O_2 to peripheral tissues.

3. CNS consequences
   Hypothermia decreases cerebral blood flow and nerve conduction velocity. Manifestations include amnesia and disorientation with mild to moderate hypothermia. Weakness, absent pupillary light reflexes and deep tendon reflex occur with severe hypothermia.

4. Renal consequences
   Mild hypothermia precipitates increased urine output ("cold diuresis"). Severe hypothermia is characterized by azotemia, oliguria, and acute tubular necrosis.

5. Hematologic consequences
   Hemoconcentration and increased blood viscosity, thrombocytopenia, and leukopenia may arise. Immunologic function is compromised predisposing the patient to infection. Circulatory failure associated with severe hypothermia may lead to disseminated intravascular coagulopathy.

E. Assessment (Table 13-2)

Physical examination is useful in estimating the severity of hypothermia. Physiologic monitoring detects life threatening changes in cardiorespiratory function. Analysis of blood specimens identifies the more subtle metabolic and hematologic complications of hypothermia.

TABLE 13-2. Assessment of the Hypothermia Victim

Site	Mild (32-35°C)	Severe (< 32°C)
Physical Examination		
Skin	•Cold, pale	•Scleremic, edematous
CNS	•Lethargic •Poor judgement •Incoordination •Slurred speech •Decreased appetite	•Obtunded, comatose, weak, flaccid, miotic pupils (< 27°C) •Nonreactive and dilated pupils (< 25°C) •Diminished deep tendon reflexes
Respiration	•Tachypnea	•Slow and shallow respirations
Cardiac	•Tachycardia	•Bradycardia, hypotension
Physiologic Monitoring		
ECG	•Sinus tachycardia	•Sinus bradycardia •T wave inversion •Prolongation of QT interval •Acute elevation of QRS-ST segment junction (Osborn or J wave) •Slow atrial fibrillation •Ventricular ectopy •Ventricular fibrillation
Hemodynamics	•↑ cardiac output •↑ systemic vascular resistance •↑ mean arterial pressure	•↓ cardiac output •↓ mean arterial pressure
Urine output	•Polyuria	•Oliguria
Laboratory Testing		
Hematologic	•↑ Hct, ↓ WBC	•Coagulopathy
Metabolic	•↓ Na^+ •↑ K^+, Glucose	•↓ pH, •↑ BUN, Amylase
X-Ray	•Ileus (<34°C)	•Ileus •Pulmonary congestion

F. Treatment (Figure 13-1)

1. Initial steps

   If the patient has a palpable pulse and is breathing, he should be moved to a warm environment. Wet or constricting clothing is removed and monitoring and assessment of the degree of hypothermia is begun. Wind currents, wet clothes, or a cold room greatly accentuate the development of hypothermia.

2. External warming for mild hypothermia

   Gentle external rewarming with warm blankets and radiant heat may be applied to achieve a rewarming rate of 1°C per hour. Intravenous fluids should be warmed through a blood warmer.

3. CPR during severe hypothermia

   If at all possible, ECG monitoring should be applied in the field to determine the presence of cardiac activity, because patients will appear comatose with barely palpable pulses. If the patient is pulseless, but has an organized cardiac rhythm on ECG, then CPR should **not** be instituted because of the risk of precipitating ventricular fibrillation. There is controversy over advisability of starting CPR in the pulseless, profoundly hypothermic patient in whom ECG confirmation of asystole or ventricular fibrillation is not possible. If CPR is initiated, it should be continued until the patient has remained unresponsive to CPR efforts despite being rewarmed to >32°C.

4. Invasive rewarming techniques

   Core rewarming is accomplished through invasive measures including assisted ventilation with heated and humidified gases, extracorporeal blood warming with partial bypass, and peritoneal dialysis with warm (43°C), potassium-free dialysate, or thoracotomy and irrigation of the heart with warm fluids.

5.   Monitoring (Table 13-3)
      ECG, core (rectal or esophageal) temperature, and urine output should be monitored in all patients. If possible, an arterial line should be placed for beat-to-beat blood pressure measurement and frequent blood sampling. Sudden cardiovascular collapse may occur because of the "afterdrop" effect in which acidotic, cold blood is mobilized from the periphery during rewarming and returned to the central circulation resulting in myocardial depression. A central venous line should not be placed until core temperature is >32°C because of possible right heart irritability. Pulmonary artery catheterization is contraindicated.

TABLE 13-3. Monitoring During Rewarming

Parameter	Expected Change
• BP (use arterial line if possible)	• ↑ in BP. Recirculation of cold blood may lead to ↓ BP.
• ECG	• Sinus or ventricular tachycardia
• Urine output	• ↑ Urine output
• Arterial blood gases	• ↑ PCO_2 when temperature ↑
• Electrolytes (esp. K^+)	• ↑ K^+
• Glucose	• ↑ or ↓
• Central venous pressure	• ↓ due to vasodilation

Hypothermia with Shallow Breathing, Coma, and Questionable Pulse

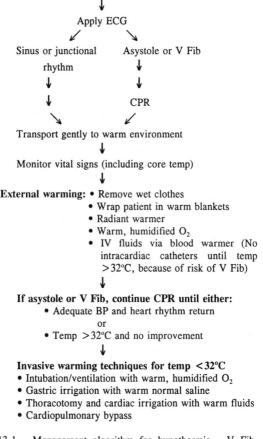

↓

Apply ECG

↙   ↘

Sinus or junctional   Asystole or V Fib
rhythm   ↓

↓   ↓

↓   CPR

↘   ↙

Transport gently to warm environment

↓

Monitor vital signs (including core temp)

↓

External warming: • Remove wet clothes
• Wrap patient in warm blankets
• Radiant warmer
• Warm, humidified O_2
• IV fluids via blood warmer (No intracardiac catheters until temp >32°C, because of risk of V Fib)

↓

If asystole or V Fib, continue CPR until either:
• Adequate BP and heart rhythm return

or

• Temp >32°C and no improvement

↓

Invasive warming techniques for temp <32°C
• Intubation/ventilation with warm, humidified O_2
• Gastric irrigation with warm normal saline
• Thoracotomy and cardiac irrigation with warm fluids
• Cardiopulmonary bypass

Figure 13-1. Management algorithm for hypothermia. V Fib, ventricular fibrillation. Temp, temperature.

II. HYPERTHERMIA (HEAT STROKE)

A. Definition

Life-threatening hyperthermia from heat stroke should be suspected when core temperature exceeds 41°C due to the inability of the body to dissipate heat.

B. Etiology

Hyperthermia occurs in the setting of environmental overheating and inability of the body to dissipate heat through sweating. A variety of congenital and chronic illnesses may predispose to the development of hyperthermia (Table 13-4). Predisposing illnesses may impair heat loss either because of abnormal ability of the skin to sweat or because of disordered CNS temperature regulation.

TABLE 13-4. Conditions Predisposing to Heat Stroke

Abnormal skin or sweating	Abnormal CNS (hypothalamic) temperature regulation
• cystic fibrosis	• tumor
• severe scleroderma	• head trauma
• ichthyosis	• meningitis-encephalitis
• ectodermal dysplasia	• stroke
• drugs: anticholinergics, beta blockers	• degenerative diseases

---

C. Pathophysiology of Heat Stroke

1. General considerations
    The pathophysiologic mechanisms of heat stroke
    are unclear, but the patient presents with
    cardiovascular collapse, stupor, and hot and dry
    skin. The body cannot dissipate heat because of
    absent sweating and peripheral vasoconstriction.

2. Infant predisposition
    Infants have a relatively large body surface area
    which allows increased conduction of heat from
    the environment.

D. Evaluation

1. Physical examination
    Heat stroke often occurs suddenly with
    temperature of 41 - 44°C (106 - 112°F). Prodromal
    signs include dizziness, headache, and confusion.
    These findings progress to prostration, coma,
    tachypnea, and shock. The skin is hot and dry.
    Children < 5 yrs of age are more likely to
    develop seizures. Irreversible brain damage
    (protein denaturation) may occur with core
    temperature >43°C.

2. Laboratory tests (Table 13-5)
    Common laboratory abnormalities during heat
    stroke include increased BUN, elevated liver
    enzymes, proteinuria, hemoconcentration, and
    leukocytosis. The ECG reveals sinus tachycardia,
    sinus arrhythmia, as well as ST and T wave
    abnormalities.

TABLE 13-5. Laboratory Abnormalities in Heat Stroke

Laboratory Test	Abnormality
• CBC	↑ Hct, ↑ WBC, ↓ platelets
• Coagulation profile	↑ PT, ↑ PTT, ↓ fibrinogen (DIC)
• Chemistry	↑ BUN, ↑ creatinine, ↑ liver enzymes, ↓ glucose, ↓ calcium, ↓ phosphate
• Urinalysis	Proteinuria
• ECG	Sinus tachycardia, sinus arrhythmia, T wave inversion, ST segment depression
• Arterial blood gas	↓ pH, ↓ pCO_2, ↓ bicarbonate (mixed metabolic acidosis and respiratory alkalosis)

E. Management (Figure 13-2)

The management of the hyperthermia patient is divided into the initial field management and the more intensive support in the emergency room and intensive care unit. Field management is devoted to airway protection of the comatose patient and intravenous hydration. Hospital management concentrates on active cooling including immersion in a cold water bath and on prevention of secondary complications such as disseminated intravascular coagulopathy (DIC) and renal failure.

Hyperthermia: Field Management

Remove from heat source
↓
Maintain patent airway and breathing with 100% O_2 in obtunded patients.
↓
Remove clothing
↓
IV hydration (Ringer's lactate 10-20 ml/kg)
↓

Hyperthermia: Hospital Management

Continue hydration with ice cold IV fluids via peripheral vein until BP and HR stable.
↓
Immersion in ice water with massage of limbs
↓
Gastric lavage with iced normal saline
↓
Sodium bicarbonate 1-2 mEq/kg for metabolic acidosis and pH < 7.2

Discontinue cooling when temp < 39° C and observe for complications
↓
DIC: fresh frozen plasma 10 ml/kg
    platelet concentrate 4 units/m² body surface area
Seizure: diazepam 0.1 mg/kg; phenytoin 10 mg/kg

Figure 13-2. Management algorithm for environmental hyperthermia (heat stroke). BP - Blood pressure; HR - heart rate.

F. Malignant Hyperthermia

1. Definition
   Malignant hyperthermia (MH) is a genetic disorder characterized by rapid increases in body temperature (1°C/5 min) secondary to uncontrolled muscle metabolism. It is triggered by volatile general anesthetics and succinylcholine. Patients with a variety of neuromuscular disorders are at increased risk for MH.

2. Management
   Specific therapy entails the prompt administration of dantrolene 2 mg/kg IV q 5 min up to maximum of 10 mg/kg after discontinuing all triggering agents. General therapy is as outlined in Figure 13-2.

G. Neuroleptic Malignant Syndrome (NMS)

NMS develops rarely after the use of major tranquilizers such as haloperidol, phenothiazines, and thiothixene. It is characterized by muscle rigidity, autonomic instability, obtundation, and hyperthermia. Management involves discontinuation of all major tranquilizers, administration of dantrolene 2 mg/kg IV, and general care as outlined in Figure 13-2.

III. NEAR DROWNING

A. Overview

Drowning is the second most common accidental cause of death after motor vehicle accidents in children. Near drowning is associated with significant morbidity. Most pediatric drowning victims are under the age of 5 and the drowning episode generally occurs during unsupervised swimming in pools, lakes, or rivers. Other risk factors include drug ingestion, epilepsy, trauma, and child abuse.

B. Pathophysiology

1. Sequential events in the drowning process
    Studies have suggested that the majority of near drowning victims go through a stage of panic and struggle to surface. This is followed by apnea and transient laryngospasm and ends in gasping respirations during which emesis and water may be aspirated.

2. Laryngospasm
    In approximately 10% of near drowning episodes, laryngospasm persists following submersion so that no aspiration pneumonia occurs.

3. Electrolyte abnormalities
    Most patients do not aspirate sufficient volumes of water to alter their electrolyte balance.

4. Pulmonary Dysfunction
    Pulmonary function and arterial blood gas derangements are common in near drowning victims. These may be transient or persistent depending on whether emesis and large volumes of water were aspirated.
    a. Laryngospasm and minimal aspiration
        Patients who have not aspirated because of laryngospasm, have transient pulmonary dysfunction. Blood gases are readily restored after assisted ventilation with supplemental oxygen.

b. Significant Aspiration

Significant aspiration pneumonia may lead to a wash-out or inactivation of surfactant causing alveolar collapse. In addition, a mediator cascade is triggered which leads to destruction of the alveolar capillary membrane and pulmonary hypertension. These patients may develop Adult Respiratory Distress Syndrome (ARDS) and require high levels of positive end expiratory pressure (PEEP) to restore normal oxygenation. In most instances, the lung injury is reversible even after significant aspiration.

5. Cerebral Anoxia

Neurologic injury secondary to anoxia is the most devastating pathophysiologic derangement in near drowning. The extent of neurologic injury is dependent on the duration of submersion and the rapidity of resuscitation. Prolonged anoxia leads to cytotoxic edema in the brain and loss of cerebral autoregulation. Cerebral edema in turn produces a rise in intracranial pressure which may lower cerebral blood flow causing further ischemia.

6. Myocardial Failure

The anoxic episode may depress myocardial function leading to shock and ultimately cardiac arrest. The resulting ischemia may produce end organ damage in the kidneys (acute tubular necrosis), in the gut (ileus and mucosal sloughing), and in the liver (ischemic hepatitis).

7. Profound Hypothermia

a. Neurologic Consequences

Submersion in very cold (< 20°C) water produces a specific sequence of pathophysiologic events. The "diving reflex" is initiated in which breathing efforts are inhibited, heart rate slows, but blood pressure is preserved. Profound vasoconstriction to non-vital organs occurs, but cerebral blood flow and metabolism may remain balanced. Thus, near drowning in very cold water may be associated with a chance for improved neurological outcome.

b. Myocardial Consequences
Myocardial contractility is depressed by hypothermia. Resuscitation may be impossible until rewarming methods have been instituted.

C. Management of Awake and Alert Patients

The survival of near drowning victims is directly related to the rapidity of rescue from the water and to the effectiveness of CPR instituted at the site of the accident.

These patients have not suffered a significant injury and primarily have pulmonary problems following their rescue.

1. Overnight observation
Pulmonary findings may evolve over the first 24 hours. Even well appearing patients should be observed overnight following near-drowning.

2. Respiratory assessment
a. Arterial blood gas: a $PaO_2 < 100$ mmHg in 60% O_2 generally requires intubation and positive end expiratory pressure support.
b. Chest X-Ray findings include: normal chest, pulmonary edema, aspiration, pneumothorax. Radiologic findings do not correlate with outcome.

3. Respiratory support
   a. PaO_2 should be maintained between 70-100 mmHg. Positive end expiratory pressure (PEEP) as high as 15-20 cm H_2O is often necessary.
   b. $PaCO_2$ should be normalized (35-40 mmHg).

4. Fluids and electrolytes
   IV fluids are administered at 2/3 the maintenance rate to limit the development of pulmonary edema (see *Chapter 5*, section VII).

5. Miscellaneous
   Routine antibiotic prophylaxis is not indicated unless contaminated water has been aspirated.

D. Management of Unconscious, Apneic Patients

These patients have experienced a cardiac arrest either at the site of the drowning, in transport, or at the hospital. Outcome is almost entirely dependent on the extent of neurologic injury. Care is supportive, and should be aimed at normalizing cardiorespiratory status. There is no evidence that neuro-resuscitation (*Chapter 15*) techniques such as barbiturates, mannitol, hyperventilation, or steroids improve outcome.

1. CPR (*Chapter 6*)

2. Hemodynamic support
   a. Invasive monitoring
      (1) Intra-arterial catheterization
      (2) Central venous catheterization
      (3) Pulmonary artery catheterization may be needed to determine preload and cardiac output in order to titrate fluid volume administration and inotropic support.

        b.   Inotrope infusions (dopamine, epinephrine) are needed frequently.

3.   Respiratory Support
Ventilatory management should be aimed at normalizing arterial blood gases (see above).

4.   Neurologic support
        a.   Associated head and neck trauma is ruled out (see *Chapter 15*).
        b.   Seizures are treated with diazepam and phenytoin.

Chapter 14
CHILD ABUSE

I. BACKGROUND

A. Epidemiology

1. Maltreatment is a highly prevalent problem. In the past two to three decades, the number of reported cases of maltreatment has risen from a few thousand to over a million per year -- about 2 per 100 US children.

2. In national surveys, from 2 to 4 percent of families report that they have at one time kicked, bit, punched, or beat up a child, or threatened a child with a deadly weapon.

3. Homicide is the fourth leading cause of death among children ages 1-4 years, ahead of heart disease, pneumonia, and meningitis.

B. Role of Medical Personnel

1. Medical personnel play an important role in detecting maltreatment and in meticulously documenting medical evidence that may lead to appropriate action and treatment for the family.

2. The approach to maltreatment is a team effort, involving social work, nursing, and medicine from within the hospital and community agencies (police, social services, prosecutors) concerned with the welfare of children and families.

II. SKELETAL TRAUMA

A. Skeletal Lesions Very Suspicious of Abuse

1. Metaphyseal tufts, periosteal thickening
   a. Location
      Most common in distal femur, proximal tibia, but also in long bones of upper extremity
   b. Radiologic appearance
      Metaphyseal injuries have appearance of tufts, chips, arcs of bone ("bucket handles"), but all are thought to be differing X-ray projections of the same lesion (fracture through diaphysis just below growth plate).
   c. Time course
      (1) Acute
          May be visible as subtle lucency along end of bone (as seen in chronic diseases such as leukemia), or possibly as apparent "chip" fracture
      (2) Subacute
          Visible after 10-14 days as repair takes place (most common scenario)
   d. Etiology
      Twisting of extremity, either directly or when trunk is shaken.

2. Rib fractures
   a. Radiologic appearance
      Usually non-displaced and thus invisible until callus formation seen at 10-14 days.
      Most frequently seen posteriorly near attachment to spine and laterally; may be obscured on standard chest films.
   b. Symptoms
      Rare, especially in infants, despite multiple fractures.

c. Etiology
Direct blows to chest and from chest
compressions, either A-P or from sides.
Rib fractures thought to be rare in CPR
except in the case of sick, premature infants
with demineralized bones.

3. Skull fractures
a. Simple, non-displaced linear skull fractures
(usually parietal) seem to be consistent with
minor household trauma (falls from beds and
chairs), although relatively infrequent given
the number of such falls.
b. Radiologic appearance
Features suggestive of greater force than
consistent with minor houusehold trauma
(and thus raising the possibility of
intentional injury) include:
(1) Fracture wider than 3 mm.
(2) Complex fracture (branching lines,
multiple fractures, involvement of
sutures).
(3) Bilateral fractures.
(4) Involvement of skull outside parietal
area.
c. Time course
Impossible to determine in skull fractures in
contrast to long bone injuries.
d. CT scan
Unreliable for detection of skull fractures,
and standard films needed if suspicion
exists.

B. Skeletal Lesions Seen in Intentional and Unintentional Injuries

1. Long bone fractures (both spiral and transverse)

    a.   Spiral fractures can happen in any setting where there is sufficient rotational force.

    b.   Transverse fractures seem to be just as common in abuse; probably caused by direct blows. Transverse fracture of the radius and ulna, for example, may be associated with raising the arm to protect the face from a blow.

    c.   Nursemaid's elbow (subluxation of radial head). Commonly found in toddlers learning to walk when child trips with arm being held extended over the head by supporting adult.

        (1)   Some children seem susceptible to repeated dislocations of the same elbow.

        (2)   Abuse could be considered if parenting problems found as well.

C.   Differential Diagnosis

1.   Minor trauma

    a.   Little biomechanical data available, but case series suggest that falls from household furniture or down moderately short flights of steps are unlikely to result in serious injury.

    b.   Falls that involve greater distances (5-6 feet or more), landing on a hard surface (concrete, steel), from a baby walker, or an adult falling on top of a child while going up and down stairs may result in more serious injury, but, still, with relatively low frequency.

2.   Skeletal disorders with increased tendency to fracture, or abnormal findings in long bones and similar radiologic appearance to traumatic injuries:

    a. osteoporosis secondary to immobility,
        prematurity, poor nutrition
    b. scurvy
    c. osteogenesis imperfecta
    d. Menkes' kinky hair syndrome
    e. rickets
    f. congenital syphilis
    g. infantile cortical hyperostosis
    h. leukemia

3. Traumatic delivery

    a. May have clavicular fractures, often along
        with brachial plexus injury
    b. Periosteal changes in diaphysis of long
        bones

D. Skeletal Surveys

1. Yield
    Greatest in children under 2-3 years of age, and
    possibly older in handicapped children with
    decreased mobility

2. X-ray survey advantages
    Less costly, more readily available, less radiation
    than bone scans, better at detecting bilateral lesions
    and fractures that may be obscured by areas of
    rapid bone growth.

3. Bone scan advantages
    Fractures detectable both earlier than radiologically
    visible and in locations which are difficult-to-see
    radiologically (ribs, hands, or feet).

4. Both may give false-negative results depending on
    technique, interpretation, and type of lesion.

III. "SHAKEN BABY" SYNDROME

A. Signs
First described as involving constellation of intracranial injuries, retinal hemorrhages, long-bone fractures in young infants (median age 6 months). More recent studies suggest that most cases probably involve striking the head against an object, as well.

B. Symptoms

Usually present with symptoms of CNS dysfunction: seizures, apnea, lethargy, vomiting. Lack of trauma history makes diagnosis difficult. May mimic primary seizure disorder, metabolic disease, spontaneous CNS bleed.

C. Evaluation

1. Retinal exam
   Retinal hemorrhages include sublaminar ("blot","pre-retinal"), flame, and dot configurations. Debate about how specific these are for trauma (vs. increased intracranial pressure), or what kinds of trauma (direct blows to head vs. forces transmitted via vasculature from chest or abdomen). Recognition of retinal hemorrhages mandates consideration of head injury vs. sepsis or metabolic disease.

2. Lumbar puncture
   Bloody fluid obtained in sepsis workup should not be assumed to be the result of a "traumatic" tap. Fluid should be spun: xanthochromic supernatant suggestive of CNS bleed.

3. Cranial imaging techniques
MRI, when available, may be more sensitive for small subdural fluid collections and for fresh parenchymal lesions than CT.

IV. ABDOMINAL INJURIES

A. General

1. Among highest mortality rates from abuse: as many as 50% of those requiring inpatient care die.

2. May be a marker for later stages of abuse within families: many children with these injuries are already known to social service system.

B. Duodenal hematoma

1. Mechanism
Blunt force compresses bowel against spine, usually producing intramural bleeding. Obstruction develops slowly (1-5 days), patients are often thought to have gastroenteritis until vomiting becomes bilious.

2. Diagnosis
Few external signs (bruises or abrasions over abdomen not often found). Oral contrast studies or CT best. Ultrasound may be useful, especially if it is available more quickly.

C. Ruptures of Major Abdominal Organs

High mortality rate. Misleading or incomplete history leads to delay in diagnosis. Altered hemodynamics are often attributed to head injury before massive blood loss recognized.

V. BURNS

A. Physiology

1. Temperature thresholds
Studies in adults suggest that temperatures below 45°C require hours to produce second or third degree burns. Above that, however, time required for burns falls by half for each °C up to about 51°C, with steeper fall-off at higher temperatures. At 53°C, time to burn is about 1.5 minutes, while at 60°C it is only a few seconds.

2. Pain sensation
Variable, but most people probably experience pain at temperatures which are safely below thresholds for rapid burns.

3. Skin characteristics
Children's skin may burn at lower temperatures because of decreased thickness or differences in vascular supply.

4. Common household sources of hot liquids and surfaces:
   a. Boiling beverages cool to 70-80°C after pouring.
   b. Electric hair curlers can have surface temperatures over 90°C when on, and some retain ability to burn for 10-15 minutes after being turned off.

B. Immersion Burns

1. Appearance caused by quick immersion in liquid that is hot enough to burn in a matter of seconds: usually no splash or run marks and sharp demarcation between burned and normal skin.

2. Stocking-glove appearance on extremities. Common pattern seen in infants is burns to buttocks and lower legs, sparing feet because of flexed knees.

3. Other spared areas may include soles of feet (thicker skin), inguinal creases (skin folded when joint flexed), or areas of buttocks that were pressed against the bottom of a tub.

4. Clothing worn at the time of immersion may alter pattern by retaining hot liquids close to the skin; may leave outline of elastic or fold of clothing.

5. Blistering and other damage to skin may not be apparent early after burn inflicted. Observation over several hours or debridement may be required before pattern clearly looks like immersion.

VI. BRUISES, BITES, AND INJURIES FROM DEADLY WEAPONS

A. Bruises

1. Color of bruise is rough indicator of age
   a. Initial: dark red or violet.
   b. 1-3 days: blue-brown.
   c. 1 week: yellow-green
   d. >1 week: light brown.
   e. Some areas of hyperpigmentation may remain for weeks.

2. Significance of bruise shape and color
   a. Dating of lesion
      (1) Progression of colors both confirms lesion as a bruise (vs. Mongolian

spots, for example) and helps date injury.

(2) Photography with color standard in frame can be important to later police work.

b. Shape

May also become more distinct with time, suggesting nature of the object that made bruise.

(1) Looped marks from cords or belts.

(2) Abraded loop may be from a rope.

(3) "Railroad tracks" from extension cord.

B. Bites

1. Significance

Can lead to identification of abuser.

2. Features

a. Type of injury

Elliptical or ovoid abrasions, bruise, or laceration. Human teeth generally crush more than lacerate. May see individual tooth marks or continuous lesion in shape of dental arch.

b. Location

Those on ears, nose, trunk, forearms may be more likely to have been inflicted for punishment.

3. Evaluation

a. Fresh marks should be swabbed for salivary residue and examined by a dentist for the possibility of making an impression or taking precise photographs.

b. Older marks can still be examined for size (adult vs. child), orientation, and readily visible dental abnormalities (deviated or

> missing teeth, gaps between central incisors).

    c.   Intercanine distances of greater than 3 cm are suggestive of adult bite.

C. Injuries from Deadly Weapons

1. Priority goes to stabilizing patient, but when possible wounds should be observed carefully before cleaning or procedures.

2. Low velocity projectiles (from small handguns, for example) crush or lacerate, while higher velocity bullets create cavitating shock waves.

3. Clothing should be examined for burns or powder residue.

4. Bullet entrance wounds appear as circular abrasion. Bruise, burn, or powder marks may also be present if bullet fired at close range (about 3 feet or less). Exit wound usually slit-like or stellate and not abraded.

VII. GENITAL INJURIES IN PREPUBERTAL FEMALES

A. Vaginal Bleeding

In the absence of other pubertal development very suggestive of trauma or foreign body.

B. External Genitalia

Injuries to posterior parts of external genitalia are more suggestive of penetrating trauma, versus anterior injuries that can be compatible with crush/straddle injury.

C. Labia Minor

1. Friability of tissues in area of posterior fourchette (where labia minor join) may be a sign of vaginitis or trauma. The area is also vulnerable to damage from instrumentation during intensive care, especially if peripheral circulation is poor.

2. Adhesions of the labia minora (usually posterior) may follow episodes of vulvitis (infectious or mechanical). There is no clear association with intentional injury. Those with total adhesion must be differentiated from vaginal agenesis (in that case urethra should be visible) or virilization.

D. Hymen

1. Configurations vary in prepubertal girls. Congenitally absent hymen seems to be very rare, but relatively few have hymen that has no opening at all if redundant folds can be sufficiently spread.

    a. Normal openings tend to be central or anterior. Rim of hymen should be fine, smooth and symmetric when labia gently retracted.
    b. Diameter of opening altered by relaxation: >6-7mm in children of school age or below may be sign of stretching from trauma, but no firm data available.
    c. Clefts in hymen posteriorly (at about 6 o'clock position) or effacing of hymenal ring (only small, rounded, thickened rim of tissue) also suggestive of injury.

E.   Rectal Injuries

1.   Debate over prevalence of serious injury -- seems higher in UK than US.

2.   Anus very expansile, possible to avoid trauma

3.   Healing seems to be rapid; within 2-3 weeks

4.   Anatomy and injuries

    a.   Anal verge injuries

        (1)   Small objects and/or well lubricated may leave no mark at all; maybe only shallow abrasion as from fingernail.

        (2)   Blood vessels may break giving rise to either localized or circumferential bruising.

        (3)   Bruise must be distinguished from normal erythema or hyperpigmentation (50-60% of black and Hispanic children, 25% of white).

        (4)   Hemorrhoids appear to be rare in children and so may be a sign of trauma (or other condition such as inflammatory bowel disease).

    b.   Shallow fissures may occur from large stool, maceration/friability, or intentional injury.

    c.   Small scars may result from fissures. May be hard to distinguish from "shiny" skin seen when perianal folds stretched. Large scars extending beyond anal verge are very likely to be caused by trauma.

    d.   Skin tags

        Seem to be relatively common in the midline; usually posterior. Outside midline raise concern for old injury.

    e.   Flattening, thickening of skin may result from repeated abrasion; underlying muscle stretched, loss of folds. Takes on "funnel shape" in extreme cases. Possibly rare in children; but found in 6/224 prepubertal suspected victims in one UK series.

f.   Persistent prominence of the anal verge may also be a sign of trauma (but may see transiently secondary to lack of relaxation)

g.   May see signs of infection (for example, genital warts).

5.   Anal canal
     Passage linking lower rectum to exterior of body; 1-3 cm long (children - adults)

a.   Trauma and infection can cause erythema and edema of anal mucosa; transient if caused by trauma.

b.   Lacerations require surgical evaluation to ensure that the walls of the canal are not penetrated.

c.   Entry of peritoneal cavity usually presents quickly.

d.   Entry of perineal space may not present until cellulitis develops.

6.   Sphincter

a.   Possible signs of abnormal dilatation
     (1) Large size (>2 cm) in absence of stool.
     (2) Asymmetry of anus when dilated.
     (3) Apparently fixed opening.
     (4) Thickening and smoothing of skin of anal verge (although smoothing alone probably normal with dilatation as muscle underlying anal verge relaxes).
     (5) Decreased "grip" on digital exam (if you believe one should be done).

b.   Signs of injury to sphincter
     (1) Acute stretching may cause anus to remain open for hours.

(2) Subsequent period of spasm if no rupture of muscles.

(3) Non-stretching injury may also be followed by spasm to "splint" tissues of anal verge.

(4) Repeated stretching can apparently lead to ability to accommodate very large objects (i.e., fisting).

VIII. MÜNCHAUSEN SYNDROME BY PROXY

A. Definition

Adult simulates, falsely reports, or induces illness in child, apparently to gain medical attention for child and family.

B. Common presentations

1. Long but vague histories of difficult to document complaints (seizures, abdominal pain) accompanied by doctor shopping and extensive, often invasive, work-ups.

2. Bleeding, hematuria, or hematemesis of an unusual nature (Table 14-1).

3. CNS abnormalities that have no ready explanation.

4. Biochemical chaos.
   Laboratory results that suggest either poisoning or adulterated specimens.

5. Sudden change in the status of a hospitalized patient, especially when the child has been getting better and discharge or decrease in the intensity of care is planned.

C. Mother Often Found to be Perpetrator

1. Often has knowledge of health care system from her own illness or employment.

2. Mother and child appear closely bonded but father often distant.

3. Mother often appears as "ideal" parent of a patient, very helpful and bonded to staff, but resists attempts to get to know her.

4. Level of denial high.
    Often refuses to acknowledge actions even when confronted with direct proof. Often good at convincing even skilled interviewers that they are normal ("sick but slick" syndrome).

D. Treatment

Usually requires obtaining proof that parent is inflicting injury before he or she is confronted with allegation of being abusive

1. Video surveillance.

2. Isolation of patient with documentation that symptoms do not occur when parent not present.

3. Laboratory tests to show that blood specimen, etc., is not from the patient or that specimens have been adulterated.

4. Careful teamwork is required to convince authorities that allegations are serious. Mortality rate from failed interventions is high.

IX. REPORTING REQUIREMENTS

A. Legal Obligations
All health care providers are obligated by law to report cases of suspected maltreatment to either the local police and/or child welfare agencies.

1. The degree of suspicion required is not specified in the law. One need not and should not wait until proof is demonstrable. On the other hand, even suspicions should be based on objective evidence and reporting may reasonably be delayed if no objective evidence yet exists.

2. Laws explicitly protect professionals who make good-faith reports of suspected maltreatment. The likelihood of adverse responses can be lessened by:

   a. Telling family about the nature of concerns, and the obligation to report, <u>before</u> the report is made.

   b. Carefully documenting the basis for concern, including verifying information given by other providers.

   c. Having the health care team reach consensus on the need for a report and letting the family know that the decision is one supported by all members of the team. This does not preclude one or more professionals remaining "neutral" and in a direct, supportive role.

TABLE 14-1. Substances and Maneuvers Creating or Simulating Illness in Victims of Munchausen Syndrome by Proxy[a]

Psychoactive drugs

Phenothiazines	Chloral hydrate
Imipramine	Methaqualone
Amitriptyline	Amphetamines
Codeine	Barbiturates

Drugs/substances altering fluid and electrolyte balance

Excessive table salt	Phenformin
Excessive water	Salicylates
Insulin	Theophylline
Furosemide	Chlorthalidone

Miscellaneous toxins

Pepper	Lye
Laxatives	Warfarin
Naphtha	

Other Mechanisms

Starvation

Suffocation

Fabricated history of previous diagnosis of serious illness

Operable cardiac disease

Various conditions

Epilepsy

Inflicted vaginal/rectal injury to produce bleeding

Altered laboratory studies

Simulation of cystic fibrosis by obtaining contaminated sputum samples, putting salt in collection for sweat test, adding fat to stool collection

Injection of contaminated material into intravenous lines

Putting parent's blood on child or in urine

Removal of blood from child's central venous line

Adapted from Wissow, LS: **Child Advocacy for the Clinician.** Baltimore: Williams and Wilkins, 1990.

Chapter 15
HEAD TRAUMA

I.   OVERVIEW

A.   Epidemiology

The central nervous system is involved in 60-70% of all trauma related injuries in children and is responsible for nearly 200,000 hospital admissions annually. Of these, 15,000 children require prolonged care and 4,000 children die because of their head injuries. Nearly 50% of these deaths occur within hours of injury. Acute and appropriate intervention may be lifesaving.

B.   Types of Injuries

Primary injury involves destruction of brain tissue at the time of the insult.

Secondary injury involves the destruction of viable, injured brain tissue by hypoxia, hypotension, and cerebral edema after the primary injury has occurred.

The goal of therapy is to prevent or limit secondary injury.

Closed or "blunt" trauma is the most common type of head injury in infants, children, and adults. In younger patients, this results in diffuse brain swelling. In adolescents and adults it results in focal or mass lesions.

If appropriately managed, the majority of head injured children are expected to have a relatively good outcome. Even children with significant head trauma may return to normal or near normal function.

II. PATHOPHYSIOLOGY

A. Intracranial Pressure (ICP)

1. Intracranial compliance
The cranium is a closed compartment filled with brain (and brain water), blood, and cerebrospinal fluid (CSF) (Figure 15-1). The space occupied by one of these components can increase initially (e.g., brain edema) without causing changes in intracranial pressure (ICP) because of compensatory reductions in the volume of other components (e.g., CSF may be squeezed out of the cranium into the spinal canal).
Once these compensatory mechanisms are exhausted, ICP will rise significantly with even small increases in the blood, CSF, or brain volume (Figure 15-2A).

2. Effects of Increased ICP
Rapid and/or sustained elevations in ICP compromise cerebral blood flow (CBF) and produce cerebral edema. The resultant cerebral ischemia produces more cerebral edema and further rises in ICP. A vicious cycle ensues. Ultimately, herniation of the brain across the tentorium or through the foramen magnum occurs. This elevated ICP may manifest itself as the **"Cushing Reflex"**, which is a triad of hypertension, bradycardia, and abnormal respirations. The presence of this reflex indicates significant compromise of blood flow to the brainstem and requires immediate therapeutic intervention.

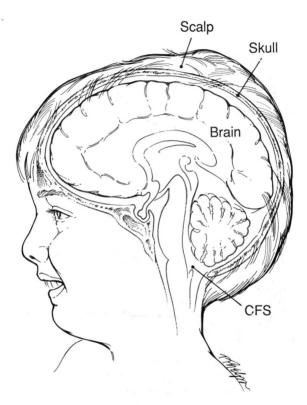

Figure 15-1. Sagittal view of the cranium. The child with head trauma is evaluated for injury to all cranial components: scalp, skull, and brain.

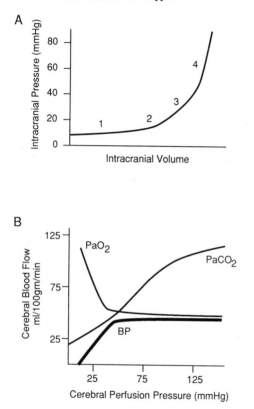

Figure 15-2. (A) Intracranial compliance curve. *Points 1-2:* Increases in intracranial volume cause only minor changes in intracranial pressure. *Points 3-4:* Even small increases in intracranial volume lead to marked rises in intracranial pressure. (B) Relationship between: (1) cerebral perfusion pressure and cerebral blood flow (CBF); (2) PaO_2 and CBF; and (3) $PaCO_2$ and CBF. See text II.B. for details.

B. **Cerebral Blood Flow (CBF)** (Figure 15-2B)

Cerebral blood flow is determined by cerebral perfusion pressure (CPP), cerebral O_2 demand ($CMRO_2$), and arterial carbon dioxide and O_2 tension.

1. Cerebral Perfusion Pressure
   CPP = MAP - ICP
   MAP is the mean arterial pressure. CPP may be reduced by either an ↑ in ICP <u>or</u> a ↓ in MAP. Under **normal** conditions, ICP is low and CPP is primarily dependent on MAP. In the **normal** brain, blood flow remains constant over a wide MAP range (50-150 mmHg). This is called **"auto-regulation"**. Auto-regulation may disappear in injured brain, and blood flow may become completely pressure dependent. A CPP greater than 70 mmHg suggests adequate CBF, whereas CPP less than 45-50 mmHg suggests marked reduction in CBF.

2. Cerebral O_2 consumption ($CMRO_2$)
   In the normal brain, CBF matches cerebral O_2 consumption. An ↑ in $CMRO_2$ (e.g., seizures, pain, excitement) will lead to an ↑ in CBF, whereas a ↓ in $CMRO_2$ (anesthesia, hypothermia) leads to ↓ CBF.

3. Arterial Carbon Dioxide Tension
   CBF is linearly related to the $PaCO_2$ over the range of 20-80 mmHg. Decreasing the $PaCO_2$ by (10 mmHg) decreases CBF by approximately 25%.

4. Arterial Oxygen Tension
   CBF remains constant at PaO_2 > 60 mmHg. With PaO_2 < 60 mmHg (O_2 saturation < 90%), CBF increases significantly.

C. Therapeutic Implications

The goals of therapy in the head injured patient are to minimize or prevent secondary brain injury utilizing the physiologic principles described above. The primary goals are to maximize delivery of O_2 and other substrate to the brain and minimize ICP. This may require manipulation of $PaCO_2$, PaO_2, MAP (blood pressure), CSF production, consciousness, and edema formation.

III. EVALUATION

A. Primary Survey

A rapid, focused and systematic physical examination (*Chapter 1*) is the most important tool in assessment of the child with head injury. **Airway, Breathing and Circulation must be quickly assessed and supported as needed.** Details of the injury should be obtained and a physical examination performed concurrently.

B. Glasgow Coma Scale (Table 15-1)

The child's neurologic status (Disability in the ABC's) can be rapidly classified according to the Glasgow Coma Scale (GCS) modified for infants and children.
A Glasgow Coma Score < 8 implies significant neurologic injury.
A Glasgow Coma Score of 9-12 is usually associated with a moderate neurologic insult.
A Glasgow Coma Score > 12 is considered a mild injury.

C. Secondary Survey (Table 15-2)

Inspection and palpation of the neck, scalp and skull must be performed. A thorough general and neurologic examination completes the assessment after the initial resuscitative management has been instituted.

TABLE 15-1. Glasgow Coma Scale

Response	Adults & Children	Infants	Points
Eye Opening	no response	no response	1
	to pain	to pain	2
	to voice	to voice	3
	spontaneous	spontaneous	4
Verbal	no response	no response	1
	incomprehensible	moans to pain	2
	inappropriate words	cries to pain	3
	disoriented conversation	irritable	4
	oriented and appropriate	coos, babbles	5
Motor	no response	no response	1
	decerebrate posturing	decerebrate posturing	2
	decorticate posturing	decorticate posturing	3
	withdraws to pain	withdraws to pain	4
	localizes pain	withdraws to touch	5
	obeys commands	normal spontaneous movement	6
Total Score			3-15

TABLE 15-2. Secondary Assessment

- Rule out associated neck injury (5-15% incidence of neck injuries in head trauma)
- X-ray or CT scan of cervical spine (including the 7th cervical vertebra)
- Evidence of basilar skull fracture (e.g., blood or CSF in ear, CSF rhinorrhea, Battle sign)
- Palpation of head and neck
- General exam

D. Neurological Examination

1. Mental Status

    Arousal, orientation, and response to parental presence.

2. Cranial Nerves

    I - Smell; *II* - Vision; *III, IV, VI* - Ocular motility, oculocephalic reflexes, pupil size, symmetry, and reactivity; *V* - Facial sensation and corneal reflex; *VII* - Facial expression and symmetry; *VIII* - Hearing and oculovestibular reflex; *IX, X* - Gag, cough, and airway protective reflexes; *XI* - Trapezius and sternomastoid movement; *XII* - Tongue movement

    a. Pupils

        The size, symmetry and reactivity of the pupils are examined (Cranial nerves III, IV, VI).

        (1) Unilateral dilation (no response to direct or consensual stimulation) of one pupil indicates compression of CN III and implies significant intracranial pathology and the possibility of impending herniation. Immediate therapy for cerebral or tonsillar herniation may be needed.

-     (2) Bilateral dilation of pupils is ominous and is due to bilateral CN III compression or severe anoxia and ischemia.
-     (3) Toxic and metabolic causes of pupillary abnormality must be excluded.

b. Extra-ocular movement

Absence or weakness of movement in any quadrant may indicate serious brain injury or orbital entrapment.

c. Oculocephalic reflexes - "Doll's Eyes" (Cranial nerves III, IV, VI)
-     (1) Do not perform in spinal injuries.
-     (2) Hold eyelids open, briskly rotate head from side to side holding briefly at endpoint (normal response - conjugate eye deviation to **opposite** side).
-     (3) Briskly flex and extend the neck (normal response-upward deviation on flexion, downward on extension).

d. Roving Eyes
-     (1) intact brainstem: slow random horizontal deviations, either conjugate or disconjugate.
-     (2) depressed brainstem: **absent** roving movement.

e. Caloric Responses (Oculovestibular reflexes)
-     (1) Inspect canals for blood, CSF, or a ruptured tympanic membrane before irrigating with ice water.
-     (2) Head 30° above horizontal.
-     (3) Small catheter (tubing from a 19 or 21 gauge butterfly IV set) placed in the external canal near the tympanic membrane.
-     (4) Slow instillation of up to 120 ml ice water.

      (5)   Observe at least 5 minutes; wait 5 minutes before irrigating opposite side

      (6)   Normal response: slow component **toward** cold and fast component **away**.

      (7)   Oculocephalic reflexes <u>can</u> be present despite **absent** cold caloric responses in patients because of preexisting vestibular disease or because of certain drugs (e.g., ototoxic agents, barbiturates, phenytoin, tricyclic antidepressants, neuromuscular blockers).

3.   Cerebellum
Coordination of voluntary movement and nystagmus

4.   Motor
Strength, tone, and posture

5.   Sensation
Pain, temperature, light touch, and two point discrimination

6.   Reflexes
Deep tendon reflexes and symmetry

IV. RADIOGRAPHIC STUDIES

Following the history and physical examination, radiographic studies may be required to make the diagnosis. Table 15-3 lists our criteria for obtaining skull films after "minor" head trauma.

TABLE 15-3. Criteria for Skull Films after Minor Head Trauma

- Age < 1 year
- Loss of consciousness >5 min
- Skull penetration
- Previous craniotomy with shunt in place
- Palpable scalp hematoma
- Skull depression
- CSF from nose or ear
- Blood in middle ear
- Battle sign (Figure 15-3B)
- Focal neurological signs

CT scans of the head (and abdomen) are required in patients with Glasgow Coma scores < 8 or who have suffered multiple trauma. These studies are obtained after the patient has been stabilized and prior to transfer to the intensive care unit. Conscious, but combative patients should be sedated and monitored to obtain the best diagnostic images possible.

V. SKULL FRACTURES

A. Linear, Nondepressed Fractures

1. No particular treatment is required.
2. Management is directed to underlying brain injury.
3. Consultation with a neurosurgeon is required only if the neurological exam is abnormal.

B. Depressed Skull Fractures

1. When a depressed skull fracture is suspected, a neurosurgical consult should be obtained.

2.   Management is primarily directed toward any underlying brain injury. Commonly, any fragment depressed more than the thickness of the skull must be surgically elevated.

C.   Compound Skull Fractures

1.   In a compound skull fracture, a direct communication exists between the scalp laceration and the cerebral substance.

2.   **Neurosurgical consultation is always indicated.** These fractures require early **operative** intervention with the elevation of the fracture, debridement of the brain, and closure of the dura.

3.   Antibiotics are usually administered.

D.   Basilar Skull Fractures

Basilar skull fractures are diagnosed on the physical examination.

1.   Raccoon eyes (Figure 15-3A)
Raccoon eyes, or circumscribed periorbital ecchymoses, are due to intraorbital bleeding from orbital roof fractures.

2.   Battle sign (Figure 15-3B)
Battle sign is an area of ecchymosis behind the pinna and suggests a mastoid fracture.

3.   CSF or bloody oto- or rhinorrhea
Bleeding or CSF drainage from the ear or nose implies a basilar skull fracture.

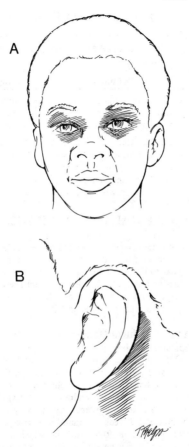

Figure 15-3. Physical signs of basilar skull fracture. (A) Raccoon eyes- periorbital ecchymoses. (B) Battle sign - ecchymosis behind the ear.

VI. CONCUSSION AND CONTUSIONS (Table 15-4)

TABLE 15-4.   Definition and Management of Concussions and
                Contusions

	Definition	**Management**
Concus-sion	Transient interruption of normal neurological function. No localizing signs; occasionally amnesia, headache, dizziness, nausea.	Observation either in the hospital or home.
Contusion	An area of bruising or microscopic hemorrhage of the brain caused by trauma, either directly (coup) or indirectly (contrecoup).	Observation in the hospital. Rarely requires surgery.

VII. INTRACRANIAL HEMORRHAGE
(Figure 15-4 A-C)

Intracranial hemorrhages can occur between the skull and the dura, between the dura and the brain substance, or in the brain parenchyma itself. These are space occupying lesions which can be classified as epidural, subdural or intracerebral hemorrhages, respectively. These lesions often continue to expand, and can produce acute increases in ICP.

A. Acute Epidural Hemorrhage (Table 15-5)

Epidural bleeding usually occurs from a tear in the middle meningeal artery. Such arterial tears are associated with linear skull fractures over the parietal or temporal bones, but occasionally may arise from a tear in the dural sinus. In children, 20% of epidural bleeds are venous in origin and may present after a lucid interval of 1-2 weeks. Epidural hemorrhage is relatively rare in children (0.5% in unselected head injuries). However, it can be rapidly fatal. This injury requires immediate surgical intervention. Secondary brain injury will occur rapidly if the hematoma is not quickly removed. If treated early, prognosis is usually good.

TABLE 15-5.	Signs and Symptoms of an Acute Epidural Hemorrhage

- Initial loss of consciousness followed by a lucid interval.
- Never entirely symptom free.
- Subsequent secondary loss of consciousness and the development of a hemiparesis on the opposite side.
- Hallmark: fixed or dilated pupil on the same side as the bleeding (in 50% of patients).
- The dilated fixed pupil may be on the side opposite from the bleeding (less common).

B.   Acute Subdural Hematoma (Table 15-6)

Subdural hematomas are usually caused by tearing of the bridging veins (Figure 15-4B). The onset of symptoms is slow. A skull fracture may be present. The underlying brain injury is often severe and the prognosis is often dismal even if the hematoma is evacuated early. Mortality with this injury is high. A subdural hematoma will not resorb and requires surgical removal.

TABLE 15-6. Signs of Subdural Hematoma

Acute Subdural Hematoma
- Fluctuations in the level of consciousness
- Hemiparesis
- Headache

Chronic Subdural Hematoma
- Similar to those of the acute
- Seizures
- Choked optic discs are more frequent

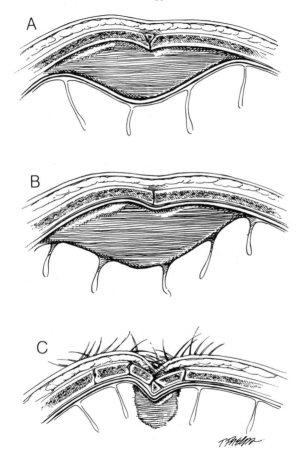

Figure 15-4. Intracranial hemorrhage. (A) Epidural hemorrhage. (B) Subdural hemorrhage. (C) Intracerebral hemorrhage.

C. Intracerebral Hemorrhage (Figure 15-4C)

Intracerebral bleeding accompanying trauma is usually small and multifocal. It is common in contused brain, directly or contrecoup. Significant intracerebral bleeding usually accompanies penetrating injuries. Late complications of these injuries depend upon the location and size of the remaining defect and include: seizure disorders, learning disabilities and other alterations in higher brain function.

VIII. PENETRATING HEAD INJURIES

These injuries require immediate neurosurgical evaluation and intervention. **Never attempt to remove a foreign body penetrating the head.**

IX. DIFFUSE CEREBRAL INJURY

Diffuse cerebral injury is the most common type of head injury in children and is found in both blunt and penetrating injury. Usually, there is no associated skull fracture or intracranial hemorrhage. Neurologic examination reveals global depression of cerebral function. Diffuse cerebral swelling is often noted on CT scan. Treatment consists of non-surgical management as described in Figure 15-5.

X. MANAGEMENT (Figure 15-5)

A. Airway - Indications to Intubate the Trachea
1. Upper airway obstruction
   Loss of pharyngeal muscle tone, inability to clear oral secretions, seizures, foreign body
2. Loss of protective airway reflexes
3. Inadequate gas exchange
   Inability to maintain $PaO_2 > 60$ mmHg (O_2 saturation $> 90\%$), respiratory failure (CO_2 retention).
4. Intracranial pressure elevation
   Hyperventilation is the single most important tool used in managing elevated ICP. CO_2 is a potent

cerebral vasodilator. Hyperventilation to reduce $PaCO_2$ to a range of 25-30 mmHg decreases cerebral blood volume and ICP. This improves perfusion and reduces edema formation.

5. Glasgow Coma Score < 8

B. Drugs to Facilitate Intubation (*Chapter 2*)

Because the larynx and trachea are very heavily innervated, intubation (and tracheal toilet) increase ICP. Various medications are used to blunt the intracranial responses and cardiovascular reflexes to intubation.

1. Thiopental (1-2 mg/kg)

Thiopental (or thiamylal) is a general anesthetic that blunts the elevation in ICP in response to intubation. It decreases brain metabolism and is used to lower elevated ICP acutely. It is a potent negative inotrope and dramatic falls in blood pressure can occur in hypovolemic patients.

2. Lidocaine (1-2 mg/kg)

Intravenous and topical lidocaine (2% solution) blunt the hemodynamic responses to intubation. Primarily used in hemodynamically unstable patients, it is often administered with fentanyl and/or midazolam.

3. Fentanyl (2-5 μg/kg)

Fentanyl is the safest opioid to use in trauma patients because it has the fewest hemodynamic side effects. Rapid IV administration can produce chest wall rigidity which makes ventilation impossible (R_x = succinylcholine or naloxone). Because pain increases ICP and many head injured patients have bone fractures, fentanyl reduces ICP by decreasing pain and blunting the response to intubation.

4. Muscle relaxants *(Chapter 2)*

Rapid paralysis of patients prevents cough-induced ICP rises, facilitates intubation, and reduces the risk of vomiting and aspiration pneumonia.

    a.   Succinylcholine (1-2 mg/kg)
        (1)   Very rapidly acting and short lived
        (2)   Contraindicated in open globe injury (see Table 2-5 for other contraindications).
    b.   Vecuronium (0.2 mg/kg)
    c.   Pancuronium (0.15-0.2 mg/kg)

C. Circulation

The brain tolerates ischemia poorly. The autoregulatory mechanisms that maintain perfusion may be damaged in head injury. The circulating blood volume, cardiac output, and blood pressure must be maintained in the normal range. Acute hypovolemic shock (*Chapter 5*) is treated with balanced salt solutions, colloid, and blood. Hypoperfusion and the use of fluids containing free water (e.g., D_5W) will worsen brain edema.

Once there is evidence of adequate perfusion (urine output > 1 ml/kg/hr), fluid restriction (1/2-2/3 maintenance requirements, *Chapter 5*) is started to minimize edema formation.

D. Diuretics

Diuretics (in combination with fluid restriction) reduce cerebral edema by enhancing the movement of brain interstitial water into the vascular spaces. There are 3 types: loop diuretics, osmotic diuretics, and carbonic anhydrase inhibitors.

1. Furosemide (1mg/kg) (loop diuretic)
   Furosemide inhibits NaCl and water resorption in the distal tubules of the kidney, reduces the intracellular accumulation of Na and water in the brain, and inhibits CSF formation.

2. Mannitol (0.25-0.5 g/kg) (osmotic diuretic)
   An osmotically active agent, mannitol draws free water from the extracellular space which is then excreted by the kidneys. Over time the overall effect is to lower ICP.

3. Acetazolamide (5 mg/kg) (carbonic anhydrase inhibitor)
    Acetazolamide prevents the recovery of Na and bicarbonate in the kidney and in the choroid plexus. This results in a diuresis of Na and water and a reduction in CSF formation.

E. Steroids

There is no clear evidence of beneficial effects of steroids in isolated head trauma. Steroids may be beneficial in spinal cord trauma (*Chapter 18* III.C.2.).

XI. OUTCOME

Children with head injuries are reported to have very promising outcomes. The amount of recovery is associated with the type of injury (focal or mass lesions vs diffuse/global injury) and severity of neurologic insult (Glasgow Coma Scale Score) and physical findings. The outcomes for different subgroups of patients are summarized in Table 15-7 (from Becker et al: J Neurosurg 47:491, 1977).

TABLE 15-7. Relationship of Coma Scale to Outcome

Coma Rating	Good recovery/ moderately disabled	Severely disabled/ vegetative	Dead
3,4	25	2	3
5,6,7	20	0	0
> 8	3	0	0

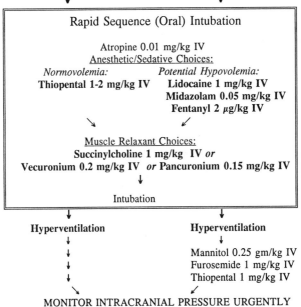

GCS >8
(Glasgow Coma Score)
↓
ABC's and Observe neurologic status closely

| **GCS <8 and** | **GCS <8 and** |
| **stable** | **impending herniation** |

| ↓ | ↓ |

Mask O₂	Bag-Mask Ventilation
Monitor Vital Signs	100% O₂ and cricoid pressure
IV Access	↓
Correct Hypovolemia	Rapid IV Access and Monitoring
↓	↓

Rapid Sequence (Oral) Intubation

Atropine 0.01 mg/kg IV
Anesthetic/Sedative Choices:

Normovolemia:	*Potential Hypovolemia:*
Thiopental 1-2 mg/kg IV	**Lidocaine 1 mg/kg IV**
	Midazolam 0.05 mg/kg IV
	Fentanyl 2 μg/kg IV

↘   ↙

Muscle Relaxant Choices:
Succinylcholine 1 mg/kg IV *or*
Vecuronium 0.2 mg/kg IV *or* **Pancuronium 0.15 mg/kg IV**
↓
Intubation

↓	↓
Hyperventilation	**Hyperventilation**
↓	↓
↓	Mannitol 0.25 gm/kg IV
↓	Furosemide 1 mg/kg IV
↓	Thiopental 1 mg/kg IV
↘	↙

MONITOR INTRACRANIAL PRESSURE URGENTLY

Figure 15-5. Algorithm for head trauma and coma.

Chapter 16
THORACIC TRAUMA

I. OVERVIEW

A. Epidemiology

1. Blunt vs. Penetrating Injury
   Greater than 90% of cases are associated with blunt mechanisms of injury (motor vehicle accidents, falls). Penetrating injuries are infrequent in children. There is a high incidence (>50%) of associated systems injuries: CNS > soft tissue and skeletal > abdominal.

2. Mortality Rates
   Overall pediatric mortality ranges 7-15%, however there is a 25% mortality in children < 6 years. Deaths occur in the early hospital course (67%). 85% of chest injuries can be managed acutely with nonoperative techniques and < 15% will require thoracotomy.

B. Pathophysiology

The compliant chest wall in children allows energy transfer to intrathoracic structures often without evidence of external chest wall injury. The mediastinum is also mobile and flexible. There is a low incidence of major vessel and tracheobronchial injury, however cardiovascular and ventilatory compromise can rapidly occur with or without mediastinal shift. Aerophagia, gastric dilatation, regurgitation and reflex ileus are common events in the post-injury phase.

C. Definition of Priorities in Thoracic Trauma

1. Highest priority: <u>Life-threatening</u>
   a. Airway obstruction
   b. Tension pneumothorax
   c. Open pneumothorax
   d. Massive hemothorax
   e. Flail chest
   f. Cardiac tamponade
2. Second priority: <u>Potentially Life-Threatening</u>
   a. Tracheobronchial injury
   b. Pulmonary contusion
   c. Myocardial contusion
   d. Traumatic aortic rupture
   e. Traumatic diaphragmatic hernia
   f. Esophageal trauma
3. Third priority: <u>Not Life-Threatening</u>
   a. Simple pneumothorax
   b. Small hemothorax
   c. Rib fracture
   d. Chest wall contusion
   e. Traumatic asphyxia
   f. Air embolism

II. LIFE THREATENING CHEST INJURY

A. Airway Obstruction

1. Definition and Pathophysiology
   Thoracic trauma may be accompanied by airway obstruction from blood, mucus, vomitus, teeth, or a foreign body. A high index of suspicion is required with closed head injury, maxillofacial or laryngeal trauma.
2. History and Physical Examination
   The physical exam is key to immediate diagnosis and treatment. Interference in ventilatory gas exchange and progressive hypoxia create a cascade

of symptoms and signs in patients with traumatic airway obstruction (Table 16-1). Diagnosis of airway obstruction is made by examination and x-rays are obtained only after the airway is secure.

TABLE 16-1. Signs and Symptoms in Acute Airway Obstruction

Agitation/confusion
Initial tachycardia
Tachypnea
Diaphoresis
Ineffective respiratory movements
Stridor
Retraction (accessory muscle recruitment)
Cyanosis
Bradycardia with progressive hypoxia

---

3. Management
   See *Chapter 2* for a detailed discussion of airway management which includes the following steps:
   a. Positioning, suctioning (clean secretions and foreign bodies)
   b. Cervical spine immobilization
   c. Supplemental oxygen administration

   If the airway cannot be maintained safely (head injury with Glasgow Coma Score ≤ 8, maxillofacial trauma), the following steps are required (Figure 16-1):

   d. Intubation
   e. Cervical spine immobilization during airway intervention
   f. Mechanical ventilation
   g. Needle cricothyrotomy may be required and is preferable to surgical cricothyrotomy in children < 12 years of age (Figure 2-12).

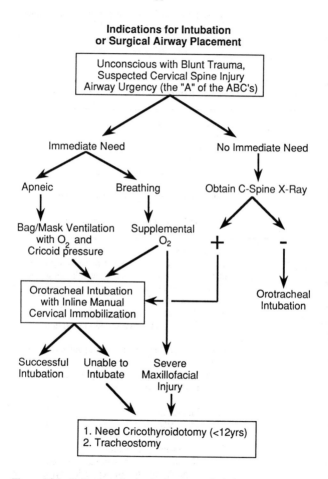

Figure 16-1. Indications for intubation or surgical airway placement.

B.   Tension Pneumothorax

1.   Definition
Accumulation of air under pressure in the pleural space.

2.   Pathophysiology
a.   Etiology
The development of a tension pneumothorax entails a communication between air passages or lung parenchyma and the pleural space. The injury results in a "closed system" such that air can enter the pleural space but cannot exit. The most common cause is high airway pressure from mechanical ventilation. Other causes include any blunt or penetrating force disrupting the tracheobronchial tree or lung parenchyma.

b.   Consequences
The expanding air space produces mediastinal shift with tracheal deviation which can interfere with central venous return and lead to decreased cardiac output. Profound respiratory distress and circulatory collapse result.

3.   History and Physical Examination (Table 16-2).

4.   Diagnostic Tests
The chest x-ray is diagnostic, but the severely compromised patient will require thoracostomy before there is time to obtain a chest x-ray.

TABLE 16-2. Signs and Symptoms with Tension Pneumothorax

EARLY: Dyspnea
Tachypnea
Unilateral chest wall movement
Decreased breath sounds on affected side
Hypertympany

LATE: Tracheal deviation
Mediastinal shift to contralateral side
Profound respiratory distress
Circulatory collapse
Distended neck veins
Cyanosis

5. Immediate Management
   a. Supplemental oxygen and secure airway (intubate if necessary)
   b. Needle thoracostomy in the midclavicular line (MCL) at 2nd intercostal space (ICS). Use a 22 gauge over-the-needle catheter in the infant and an 18 gauge over-the-needle catheter in an older child. After sterile preparation of the skin, the catheter is advanced just beyond the rib margin into the pleural space whereupon the needle is removed and the catheter is advanced further. The catheter is connected to a 20 ml syringe and a 3-way stopcock and air is evacuated.

6. Definitive Management
   A chest tube is placed in the 5th ICS just lateral to the nipple at a point between the anterior and midaxillary line (Figure 16-2). After placement the chest tube is connected to a pleurevac and suction (Figure 16-3).

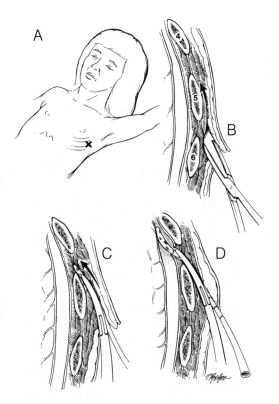

Figure 16-2. Steps in chest tube placement. (A) Sterile prep and local anesthesia to the 5th intercostal space between the anterior and midaxillary line. (B) 2 cm horizontal skin incision followed by blunt dissection with a hemostat just above the rib. (C) Chest tube is clamped between the teeth of the hemostat and (D) advanced into the pleural space. The incision is then closed and a dressing applied to stabilize the tube.

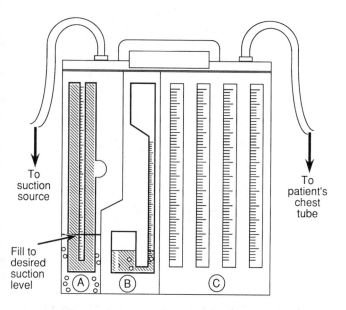

Figure 16-3. Chest tube collection system.
(A) Fill suction control chamber to desired level with sterile water.
Connect tubing from this chamber to suction source (bubbling denotes
suction). (B) Fill water seal chamber to 0 cm level with sterile water
(bubbling denotes air leak). (C) Connect tubing from collection
chamber to chest tube.

C. Open Pneumothorax (Sucking Chest Wound)

1. Definition
   There is a loss of a portion of the chest wall with an opening greater than the diameter of the airway. This permits air to pass in and out through the defect with each breath.

2. Pathophysiology
   The open pneumothorax is associated with penetrating trauma. Immediate equilibration of the intrathoracic and atmospheric pressures eliminates effective ventilation of the lung with resultant hypoxia. Mediastinal shift can occur leading to reduction in venous return.

3. History and Physical Examination
   Examination shows an obvious chest wall defect with air movement to and from the wound, along with signs and symptoms of acute respiratory distress.

4. Initial Management
   The chest wound is covered with a sterile, overlapping dressing which is taped in place on 3 sides to allow air to escape but not enter. This converts the "open" pneumothorax to a "closed" pneumothorax. The patient must be observed closely for signs of tension pneumothorax which may develop if the dressing becomes completely occlusive preventing the escape of air.

5. Definitive Management
   Tube thoracostomy in the 5th intercostal space, just lateral to the nipple, between anterior and midaxillary line (Figure 16-2). There may be a need for exploratory thoracotomy, if tracheobronchial injury exists.

D. Massive Hemothorax

1. Definition
   Blood collection >20 ml/kg in the pleural cavity indicates the presence of a massive hemothorax.

2. Etiology
   Massive hemothorax can occur in both blunt and penetrating chest trauma. It is a known complication of subclavian or internal jugular vein cannulation.

3. Pathophysiology
   Ventilatory insufficiency and hypovolemic shock develop as a result of hemothorax. Mediastinal shift exacerbates the cardiovascular compromise from hypovolemia.

4. History and Physical Examination
   a. Cardiorespiratory signs
      Signs and symptoms are identical to those of tension pneumothorax. Signs of respiratory distress usually precede evidence of poor perfusion. Thus, hemothorax may be overlooked in the intubated and mechanically ventilated patient until significant blood loss has produced hypovolemic shock. A high index of suspicion for hemothorax should be maintained in patients with a compatible history.
   b. Chest wall protuberance in infants
      The compliant infant chest wall may protrude on the affected side in the face of a large hemothorax. The subcostal region is particularly useful to detect this asymmetry.

5. Diagnostic Tests
   Chest x-ray only confirms the clinical diagnosis.

6. Initial Management
   a. Secure airway
   b. Ventilate/oxygenate

      c.   Fluid (crystalloid and blood) resuscitation for volume restoration.

      d.   Tube thoracostomy (Figure 16-2) with the chest tube angled posteriorly.

7.   Definitive Management
If blood loss continues (>2-4 ml/kg/hr x 4 hrs or >10% of blood volume), definitive thoracotomy is necessary.

E.   Flail Chest

1.   Definition
Segment of chest wall lacks bony continuity with the remaining thoracic cage.

2.   Epidemiology
The flail chest is associated with violent blunt trauma, multiple rib fractures, and underlying pulmonary parenchymal injury (contusion). Flail chest is unusual in infants and toddlers. The incidence increases with age.

3.   Pathophysiology
Ventilation perfusion (V/Q) mismatch in the contused lung leads to hypoxia. Flail segment responds to changes in intrathoracic pressure rather than to the action of the respiratory muscles. During spontaneous breathing the flail segment moves inward with the fall of intrathoracic pressure on inspiration. Conversely, the normal portions of the chest wall are pulled outward by the action of the respiratory muscles. Thus, there is paradoxical breathing. Children tolerate postero-lateral flail segments poorly, as this interferes significantly with diaphragmatic excursion.

4.   History and Physical Examination

      a.   Inspection
Flail chest is apparent on inspection and the paradoxical movement of the flail segment is pathognomonic. Effective ventilation is not possible because of the uncoordinated

        movement of the thorax. The patient develops signs of respiratory distress.

    b.   Palpation

        Paradoxical chest wall motion is also apparent on palpation of the chest wall.

        Rib fractures and crepitus are frequently palpable.

5.   Diagnostic Tests

    a.   Arterial blood gas is used to confirm inadequate ventilation ($PCO_2 > 40$ mmHg).

    b.   Chest x-ray reveals rib fractures and the pulmonary contusion.

6.   Management - Internal Stabilization

    Internal stabilization is accomplished with endotracheal intubation and mechanical ventilation with positive end-expiratory pressure (PEEP). The positive intrathoracic pressure throughout the respiratory cycle prevents inward motion of the flail segment during a spontaneous inspiration. The level of PEEP may have to be raised for large flail segments with severe underlying pulmonary contusions.

7.   IV Fluid Administration

    After resuscitation, crystalloid administration is restricted, because overhydration can worsen the pulmonary contusion.

8.   Analgesia

    Either regional or narcotic analgesia is needed to prevent splinting on the affected side.

F.   Cardiac Tamponade

1.   Definition

    Cardiac tamponade is the compression of the heart produced by accumulation of blood under pressure in the confined space of the pericardial sac.

2. Etiology

Tamponade is more often the result of penetrating rather than blunt trauma. Tamponade may also occur after thoracic or cardiac surgery and as a complication of central venous line placement. Infectious pericarditis is the major nontraumatic cause of tamponade in children.

3. Pathophysiology

The pressure in pericardial space increases rapidly and exceeds intracardiac pressure. This results in decreased filling of the heart and decreased cardiac output. The rise in ventricular end diastolic pressure produces systemic and pulmonary venous congestion. Right atrial, right ventricular, pulmonary artery diastolic, and pulmonary capillary wedge pressures are equalized.

4. History and Physical Examination

Physical examination shows narrowed pulse pressure, muffled heart tones, and distended neck veins. The diagnosis should be strongly suspected in the face of:

a. Rising central venous pressure.
b. Lowered systolic BP initially, followed by lowered mean arterial pressure.
c. Pulsus paradoxus - >10 mmHg fall in systolic BP during inspiration.

5. Ancillary tests

Echocardiogram reveals an echogenic space between pericardium and epicardium. Chest x-ray shows widened cardiac and mediastinal shadows. **Do NOT delay therapy in the symptomatic patient in order to obtain ancillary tests!**

6. Management- Airway, Breathing, and Circulation

Standard resuscitative measures are employed

including intubation and ventilation with 100% O_2 and intravenous fluid and blood administration.

7.   Pericardiocentesis (See Figure 16-4)
     Immediate subxiphoid pericardiocentesis is indicated in the patient with evidence of hypotension, systemic venous congestion, and a compatible history. A minimum of ECG and blood pressure monitoring is mandatory. Sterile prep is used in all patients. If time permits, include sterile drapes and local anesthesia in the conscious patient. A 3 inch, 22 gauge spinal needle is used in infants, whereas older children receive a 6 inch, 16 or 18 gauge over-the-needle catheter. After a small skin incision (16 gauge straight needle or a #11 scalpel blade), the spinal needle or over-the-needle catheter is attached to a 20 ml syringe with a 3-way stopcock and inserted to the left of the xiphoid process. It is advanced at a 45° angle toward the left scapular tip. Blood is aspirated once the pericardium is entered. If the needle is advanced too far (into myocardium), an injury pattern is noted on ECG consisting of marked ST-T wave changes and widened QRS complexes. Premature ventricular contractions may also appear. The needle should be withdrawn slowly until the baseline ECG pattern returns, and blood aspiration is attempted again. Pericardial blood can be distinguished from intracardiac blood by its failure to clot due to the fibrinolytic properties of the pericardium. Following pericardiocentesis the patient is observed closely for recurrent tamponade and repeated aspirations may be needed during transport to operating room.

8.   Thoracotomy
     Ongoing hemorrhage into the pericardial sac requires thoracotomy to drain the pericardium and repair the bleeding site.

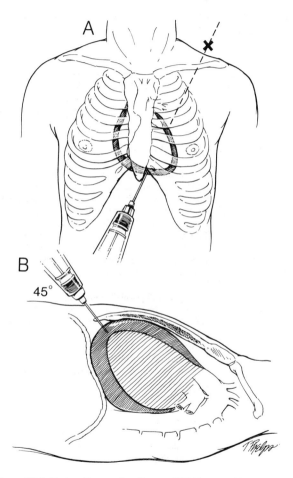

Figure 16-4. Pericardiocentesis. See text II.F.7. (page 324).

III. POTENTIALLY LIFE-THREATENING CHEST INJURY

A. Overview
The potentially life-threatening chest injuries are associated with damaged intrathoracic structures. These injuries are often missed during primary survey. The diagnosis is obtained in the secondary survey, after diagnostic and therapeutic intervention.

B. Tracheobronchial Injury

1. Presentation and Pathophysiology
   Blunt trauma injuries occur within one inch of the carina and the diagnosis can be subtle. Penetrating trauma is more overt. Pneumothorax develops with a persistent air leak after chest tube placement. Tension pneumothorax with mediastinal shift may be present. In addition, there is partial upper airway obstruction. Approximately 50% of deaths from this injury occur within one hour.

2. History and Physical Examination
   History is important in making the diagnosis, particularly in patients with blunt trauma. External evidence of trauma may not be obvious. Signs include:
   a. Labored breathing
   b. Signs of tension pneumothorax (Table 16-2)
   c. Hemoptysis
   d. Subcutaneous emphysema

3. Diagnostic Tests
   The diagnosis is suggested by persistent air leak from the chest tube. Bronchoscopy usually confirms the diagnosis.

4. Initial Management
   a. Intubation is necessary to ensure adequate oxygenation and ventilation.
   b. Chest tube placement is required, and often a second chest tube is necessary to overcome a large air leak.

5. Definitive Management
   Patients without major anatomic distortion of the tracheobronchial tree will usually heal with just supportive care. Large paratracheal hematoma requires surgical intervention.

C. Pulmonary Contusion

1. Definition
   Blunt or penetrating forces to the chest produce laceration of lung tissue and interstitial hemorrhage. It is the most common parenchymal injury after thoracic trauma.

2. Pathophysiology
   a. Ventilation/perfusion mismatch results in hypoxia.
   b. The contusion may progress to Adult Respiratory Distress Syndrome with severe hypoxemia (*Chapter 4*).
   c. Contusion may be complicated by aspiration of gastric contents, pneumothorax, or flail chest.

3. History and Physical Examination
   The initial physical exam may demonstrate hemoptysis, pleuritic pain, and labored breathing or there may be only minimal signs.

4. Diagnostic Tests
   A high index of suspicion is necessary. The diagnosis is confirmed by chest x-ray which

reveals infiltrates in lung fields usually several hours after resuscitation has been completed.

5. Management
   a. Standard Airway, Breathing, Circulation resuscitation measures.
   b. Supplemental oxygen by face mask may be sufficient in many cases.
   c. Avoid overhydration.
   d. Intubation and mechanical ventilation with PEEP is employed for patients with severe hypoxia (hypoxic on $>50\%$ O_2 by non-breathing face mask).
   e. Atelectasis is treated with chest physiotherapy.

D. Myocardial Contusion

1. Definition
   Myocardial contusion consists of a cardiac muscle injury secondary to blunt traumatic forces.
2. Pathophysiology
   The lesion involves a disruption of myocardial blood flow with subsequent myocardial ischemic injury. There exists a rare potential for infarction.
3. History and Physical Examination
   History of injury is important as physical exam can be unremarkable. Occasionally, there is visible evidence of sternal or chest wall contusion, or palpable rib fractures. Rarely, a new heart murmur can be identified.
4. Diagnostic Tests
   a. Abnormalities on the ECG (ischemic changes, premature atrial or ventricular contractions, other arrhythmias)
   b. Possible elevation of cardiac isoenzymes (CPK-MB)

5. Management
   a. Insure adequate airway and oxygenation.
   b. Continuous cardiac monitoring for ischemia, arrhythmias.
   c. Follow-up ECGs.
   d. Serial cardiac isoenzymes.
   e. Baseline echocardiogram if ECG and cardiac enzyme abnormalities are detected.
   f. In the absence of myocardial infarction the risk for long-term cardiac disability is nil.

E. Traumatic Aortic Rupture

1. Definition
   Traumatic aortic rupture entails a laceration of aorta at or distal to ligamentum arteriosum just beyond the take-off of the left subclavian artery.

2. Pathophysiology
   Tremendous force is associated with the mechanism of injury such as deceleration from high-speed motor vehicle injuries or falls from great height (i.e., plane crash). 90% of victims are dead in the field from exsanguination. Those who survive transport to a hospital have continuity of aorta maintained by an intact adventitial layer.

3. History and Physical Examination
   History of a motor vehicle accident or a fall from great height should suggest the diagnosis. Hypotension results from blood loss into the contained hematoma around the aorta.

4. Diagnostic Signs (See Table 16-3)

TABLE 16-3.	Diagnostic Signs of Traumatic Aortic Rupture

- Widened mediastinum
- Fracture of 1st and 2nd ribs
- Obliteration of the aortic knob
- Deviation of the trachea to the right
- Presence of apical pleural cap (effusion)
- Depression of the left mainstem bronchus (140° from the tracheal midline)
- Left pleural effusion
- Elevation and shift to right of the right mainstem bronchus
- Obliteration of aorticopulmonary window

DEFINITIVE DOCUMENTATION BY AORTOGRAM

5. Management

Any patient with a compatible history and a widened mediastinum on chest x-ray should be strongly considered for angiography to rule out traumatic aortic rupture. Once the diagnosis is confirmed, immediate thoracotomy is undertaken with resection of the injured area and direct repair, usually with a graft prosthesis.

F. Traumatic Diaphragmatic Hernia

1. Definition

Traumatic diaphragmatic hernia consists of large radial tears in the left hemidiaphragm following blunt trauma which allow immediate herniation of abdominal contents into the chest. Penetrating trauma produces small tears and minimal herniation.

2. Pathophysiology
   a. Herniated abdominal contents may cause mediastinal shift and acute respiratory insufficiency.
   b. There is a 10-25% incidence of associated intra-abdominal injury.

3. History and Physical Examination
   a. Tachypnea
   b. Displaced heart impulse on cardiac exam
   c. Audible bowel sounds in the chest

4. Diagnostic Tests
   a. Chest x-ray may be misinterpreted as left hemidiaphragm elevation, acute gastric distention or subpulmonic hematoma.
   b. A definitive diagnosis is made by noting displacement of a nasogastric tube into an intrathoracic stomach.

5. Management
   a. Airway, Breathing, Circulation.
   b. If assisted ventilation is needed, the patient should be rapidly intubated, because prolonged bag-mask ventilation will lead to gastric inflation and lung compression.
   c. The stomach is decompressed with an oro- or nasogastric tube to improve ventilation.
   d. Operative Management
      The acute traumatic diaphragmatic hernia should be repaired.

G. Esophageal Trauma

1. Definition
   Penetrating trauma (missiles or instrumentation) to the chest or blunt trauma to upper abdomen (crush) produce a perforation or linear tear in the esophagus.

2. Pathophysiology
Linear tear in lower left esophagus permits leakage of gastric contents into the mediastinum with early onset of mediastinitis and later rupture into the pleural space producing empyema.

3. History and Physical Examination
The clinical picture is identical to the post-emetic esophageal perforation: "Boerhave's syndrome." Signs (often delayed):
   a. Fever
   b. Tachycardia
   c. Friction rub
   d. Shock
   e. Substernal or epigastric pain out of proportion to injury

4. Diagnostic Tests
   a. Chest x-ray reveals left mediastinal air.
   b. Gastrograffin swallow demonstrates extravasation of dye into the mediastinum.

5. Management
   a. Airway, Breathing, Circulation.
   b. Operative Management
   Thoracotomy with wide drainage of pleural space and mediastinum is undertaken to prevent empyema and mediastinal abscess formation. If feasible, the esophageal tear is repaired with a patch. If repair is not feasible, the stomach is transected to allow diversion of the esophagus and proximal stomach. Gastrostomy is placed in the distal stomach segment for feeding.

IV. NON-LIFE-THREATENING CHEST INJURY

A. Simple Pneumothorax

1. History and Physical Examination
   a. History of blunt or penetrating chest trauma

      b.   Hyperresonance on percussion

      c.   Decreased breath sounds

2.   Diagnostic Tests

Chest x-ray reveals a radiolucent shadow between the rib margin and the lung parenchyma. Rib fractures should be excluded on chest x-ray.

3.   Management

Chest tube drainage to underwater seal is mandatory before the patient is transported out of the emergency room or before induction of general anesthesia for repair of other injuries (See under "Tension Pneumothorax" and Figures 16-2 and 16-3).

B. Simple Hemothorax

1.   History and Physical Examination

      a.   History of blunt or penetrating chest trauma

      b.   Dullness on percussion

      c.   Decreased breath sounds

2.   Diagnostic Tests

The decubitus view of the chest x-ray documents a radio-opaque fluid layer between the rib margin and the lung parenchyma.

3.   Management

Chest tube drainage. (See under "Massive Hemothorax" and Figures 16-2 and 16-3.)

C. Rib Fractures

1.   History and Physical Examination

      a.   Palpable crepitus

      b.   Rib deformity

      c.   Asymmetrical chest wall movement

      d.   Pain leads to splinting of thorax with impaired ventilation.

      e.   Fracture of 1st-2nd ribs carries a risk for significant intrathoracic injury.

       f.   The middle ribs (5-9) are most commonly injured.

2.   Diagnostic Tests

Chest x-ray confirms the presence of rib fractures and excludes other chest injuries.

3.   Management

    a.   Supplemental O_2

    b.   Pulmonary toilet

    c.   Avoid atelectasis and pneumonia by providing analgesia and encouraging deep breathing.

    d.   Analgesia is achieved with narcotics (*Chapter 10*) or regional nerve blocks (e.g., intercostal nerve blocks).

D.   Chest Wall Contusion

1.   History and Physical Examination

There is obvious evidence of blunt external trauma (soft tissue injury, abrasions, lacerations).

2.   Diagnostic Tests

Chest x-ray is used to exclude other intrathoracic injury.

3.   Management

    a.   Local wound care

    b.   Deep breathing exercises to avoid atelectasis and pneumonia

E.   Traumatic Asphyxia

1.   Definition

This is an unusual injury which is more common in children because of their compliant chest wall. A crushing blunt force produces a compressive chest injury which increases intrathoracic pressure. Increased intrathoracic pressure is transmitted through the superior vena cava to the head and neck such that blood dissects through the walls of venules.

2. History and Physical Examination
   a. Head, neck, upper torso cyanosis or petechial hemorrhages
   b. Conjunctival/retinal hemorrhages
   c. Signs of respiratory distress
   d. CNS depression secondary to rapid increase in intracranial pressure.
3. Diagnostic Tests
   The diagnosis is made by physical examination.
4. Management
   a. Airway, Breathing, Circulation.
   b. Intubation and mechanical ventilation for associated pulmonary contusion and Adult Respiratory Distress Syndrome.
   c. Rule out brain injury with CT scan of brain.
   d. Consider intracranial pressure monitoring and therapy (*Chapter 15*).

F. Air Embolism

1. Definition
   A communication between the skin opening and a central vein or between a bronchus and a pulmonary vein leads to embolization of air to the heart.
2. History and Physical Examination
   a. Usually, a history of penetrating trauma with exposed veins in the head or neck.
   b. "Mill-wheel" murmur
   c. Cardiovascular collapse may develop because of obstruction of the ventricular outflow tract with air.
   d. Signs of respiratory distress may develop because embolic obstruction of the pulmonary vascular bed leads to pulmonary congestion.
   e. Focal neurologic deficits may arise because of air embolization to the cerebral circulation.

3. Diagnostic Tests
   The diagnosis is usually made by history and physical examination. In the previously monitored patient, air embolism is suggested by a sudden fall in the endtidal CO_2 tension or by a change in pitch of a doppler ultrasound detector on the chest over the heart.

4. Management
   a. Airway, Breathing, Circulation.
   b. Ventilate patient with 100% O_2.
   c. Cover open wounds with saline soaked pads
   d. Immediately position patient in Trendelenburg position with the left side down.
   e. If a right atrial catheter is in place, aspiration of air may be attempted.

V. RESUSCITATIVE THORACOTOMY

Often conventional resuscitative tactics fail for acute cardiopulmonary arrest after thoracic trauma and thoracotomy for open-chest cardiac massage must be considered. Indications include:

A. Blunt injury in which patient arrives with vital signs and acutely deteriorates.

B. All exsanguinating penetrating chest injuries.

Chapter 17
ABDOMINAL TRAUMA

I. OVERVIEW

A. Abdominal Injury is a Major Cause of Accidental Death in Children.

1. Blunt injuries cause 90% of abdominal trauma.
2. Abdominal injury usually occurs with other multiple injuries involving the head, skeleton and chest.

II. BLUNT INJURY

A. Pathophysiology

1. Injury results from energy transfer from compressive/crushing forces or from rapid deceleration.
2. The liver and spleen are most commonly injured (solid organs).
3. Hollow visceral (bowel) injuries are often insidious in presentation.
4. The bowel (duodenum > jejunum > ileum > colon) and pancreas are vulnerable to forces from rapid deceleration with seat belt injuries.
5. Injuries to the kidney result in a spectrum of diagnoses which vary from a simple contusion of the kidney to perinephric hematoma to vascular disruption (rare).
6. Lower urinary tract injuries occur in association with pelvic fractures.

B. Evaluation (Table 17-1)

1. Abdominal injury should be suspected in any child with polytrauma and signs of hemorrhagic shock.

2. Abdominal injury is ruled out in any child with CNS injury whose abdominal exam is unreliable.
3. Acute gastric distention occurs frequently.
4. Insertion of an orogastric tube is mandatory to adequately examine the child's abdomen.

TABLE 17-1. Evaluation of the Child with Suspected Abdominal Trauma

---

LOOK

- External signs of soft tissue injury on the anterior abdominal wall (bruises, abrasions, lacerations, seat belt markings)
- Lateral flank bruising, hematoma
- Perineum - blood at urethral meatus
- Scaphoid abdomen
- Abdominal distention or masses

LISTEN

- Presence or absence of bowel sounds
- Bowel sounds are often present despite intra-abdominal injury

PALPATE

- Superficial and deep palpation
- Distinguish voluntary response (guarding) from involuntary response (peritoneal irritation)
- Anterior (splenic, hepatic) anatomic quadrants
- Flanks (kidneys)
- Lower suprapubic region - rock pelvis to insure stability
- Perineum/anorectal region as well as urethral meatus for injury

---

C. Diagnosis

1. Abdominal Radiography

   a. Supine abdominal and pelvic film
   b. Cross table lateral film
   c. Documentation of the following

      (1) High diaphragm position suggestive of subdiaphragmatic fluid collection.
      (2) Ileus pattern with diffuse bowel dilatation suggestive of aerophagia or intraperitoneal blood.
      (3) Extraluminal intraperitoneal air or fluid suggestive of visceral perforation.
      (4) Obliteration of retroperitoneal fat lines suggestive of retroperitoneal hematoma.
      (5) Rib or spine fractures.

2. Computed Tomography (CT)

   a. Over the last decade CT scanning has become state of the art imaging for blunt abdominal trauma.

      (1) Effective for evaluation of the retroperitoneum (pancreas).
      (2) CT is important particularly for non-operative management of solid organ injury (spleen, liver, kidney).
      (3) With IV water soluble contrast, renal function can be ascertained.
      (4) Optional use of oral contrast for evaluation of hollow viscus injury (stomach, duodenum, small and large bowel).

3. Intravenous pyelography (IVP)/
    Urethrocystography (UCG)

    a. Any blood at urethral meatus <u>requires</u>
        urethrocystography to exclude lower urinary
        tract injury before Foley catheter placement.

    b. UCG is used in extensive pelvic fractures.

    c. Hematuria (microscopic or gross) needs
        assessment either by IVP or CT with
        contrast.

4. Peritoneal lavage

    a. With blunt trauma, peritoneal lavage
        provides rapid assessment of an **unconscious**
        patient for intra-abdominal blood or bowel
        perforation.

    b. Indications

        (1) Patient with polytrauma whose other
             injuries require immediate operative
             intervention (ie., head or skeletal
             injury).
        (2) Unavailability of CT.
        (3) Normal CT study in a child with a
             presumed hollow viscus (bowel)
             injury.

D. Management (Figure 17-1)

1. Initial (primary survey)

   a. ABC's
      (1) Secure airway.
      (2) Supplemental oxygen or mechanical ventilation.
      (3) Large bore IV access in the upper extremities, jugular veins or subclavian veins for fluid resuscitation.
   b. Blood sent for type and cross match, CBC, amylase, electrolytes.
   c. Immediate orogastric tube placement for decompression; inspect for blood.
   d. Urinary output monitoring
      (1) Index for adequacy of resuscitation
      (2) Assess for blood

2. Definitive (secondary survey)

   a. Further diagnostic studies such as contrast CT or IVP may be indicated after patient has been stabilized.
   b. Patients with head injury and suspected abdominal injury need head and abdominal CT scans.
   c. Non-operative management protocols for splenic, hepatic, renal injury may be indicated.
   d. Operative intervention if patient becomes hemodynamically unstable.

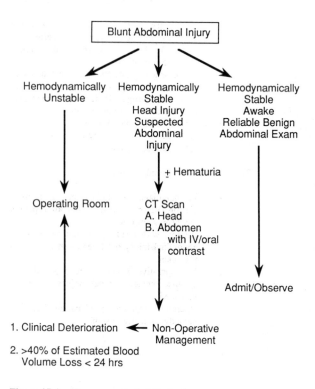

Figure 17-1. Management of abdominal trauma.

III. PENETRATING TRAUMA

A. Pathophysiology
1. Mechanisms of injury associated with gunshot wounds and stab injuries.
2. Virtually all intra-abdominal organs are at risk for injury.
3. High incidence of hollow visceral (bowel) injury.
4. Manifestations of hemorrhagic shock.

B. Evaluation (LOOK, LISTEN, PALPATE)
With history of penetrating injury, one assumes intra-abdominal injury until proven otherwise.
1. Thorough inspection for entrance and exit wound sites.
2. Presence or absence of bowel sounds may not reflect the magnitude of injury.
3. Evidence of peritoneal signs suggesting intra-abdominal blood, bowel contents.

C. Laboratory Diagnosis
Absolute minimal studies required before exploratory surgery:
1. Supine abdominal film
2. Lateral cross table view (location of foreign body)
3. Chest x-ray
4. Single injection excretory urogram

D. Management
1. Initial
   a. ABC's
      (1) Secure airway.
      (2) Supplemental oxygen or mechanical ventilation.
      (3) Large bore IV access in the upper extremities, jugular veins or subclavian veins for fluid resuscitation.

        b.   Blood sent for type and cross match, CBC, amylase, electrolytes.

        c.   Immediate orogastric tube placement for decompression; inspect for blood.

        d.   Urinary output monitoring.

            (1)   Index for adequacy of resuscitation.

            (2)   Assess for blood.

        e.   Minimal diagnostic studies as above.

2.   Definitive - abdominal exploratory surgery

Chapter 18
ORTHOPAEDIC INJURIES

I. OVERVIEW

Differences in the child's bone lead to unique injuries. Musculoskeletal injuries occur in approximately 40% of pediatric multiple trauma victims.

II. DIFFERENCES IN THE CHILD'S SKELETON

A. Fracture Patterns
Cortex of the child's bone is porous and less brittle than the adult bone, so that unique fracture patterns, rarely seen in adults, occur:
1. Plastic deformation - a bend in the bone without a fracture.
2. Greenstick fracture - a fracture of one cortex under tension while the contralateral cortex remains intact.
3. Torus fracture - a fracture with buckling of one cortex in compression while the contralateral cortex is undamaged.

B. Bone Healing
Healing after a fracture in children is characterized by: rapidity, rare nonunion, and good remodeling potential. However, growth plate disturbances are possible which may cause late deformity.

C. Growth Plate
Ligaments are stronger than bone or growth plate in children (Figure 18-1). Thus, dislocations and sprains are relatively uncommon, while growth plate disruption and bone avulsion are more common in children. Growth plate injuries are described using the Salter classification (Figure 18-2).

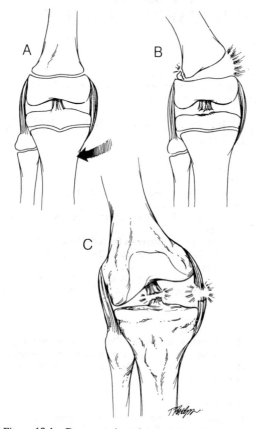

Figure 18-1. Demonstration of the relative strength of ligaments in children. (A) Following a valgus force (arrow) to the knee, the child's knee may sustain: (B) growth plate injury or cruciate avulsion from bone. (C) In an adult, the same injury would cause rupture of one or both ligaments.

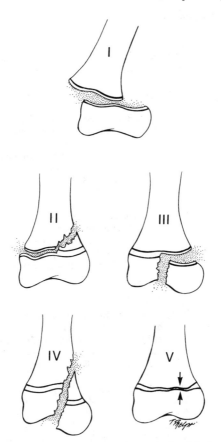

Figure 18-2. Salter classification of growth plate injuries.
I. Fracture along but not across plate; II. Fracture along plate with metaphyseal extension; III. Fracture into joint; IV. Fracture across plate and joint; V. Crush injury to plate without obvious fracture.

D. Evaluation

1. History
   If the victim is conscious, a history is obtained to determine sites of pain.

2. Neurologic Examination

   a. Nerve injury classification
      (1) Neuropraxia - a physiologic but not anatomic disruption.
      (2) Axonotmesis - axonal disruption, but not complete transection.
      (3) Neurotmesis - complete nerve transection.

   b. Common sites of nerve injury
      (1) Posterior hip dislocation
      (2) Distal humerus fracture
      (3) Severe shoulder injuries
          usually correlate with amount of bone displacement

   c. Rapid exam method
      A rapid neurologic examination is focused on motor strength including active flexion and extension of each major joint. Sensation should be tested on the dorsal and volar surfaces of each limb segment.

3. Skeletal Examination
   The cervical spine remains immobilized until fracture is ruled out. The spine is palpated for tenderness and swelling. Pelvic stability is assessed by lateral compression. The extremities are examined for swelling and ecchymoses as signs of possible fractures or dislocations. In the absence of obvious fractures, passive flexion and extension are performed on all extremities.

4. Vascular Examination

Vascular integrity must be ensured in every patient with musculoskeletal trauma. Fractures and dislocations around the elbow and knee are susceptible to vascular injury because arteries are tethered to bones at these sites. Poor peripheral pulses and slow capillary refill suggest vascular injury. Pain on passive stretch and tense swelling in a fascial compartment in addition to signs of vascular insufficiency suggest acute compartment syndrome.

5. X-rays

Areas indicated by abnormal physical findings (swelling, displacement, etc.) should be x-rayed. Specialized studies (computerized tomography, magnetic resonance imaging, or angiography) are obtained after consultation with an orthopedic surgeon. Orthopaedic surgery should be called early to help coordinate proper imaging and management.

III. SPECIFIC INJURIES

A. **Elbow** (Figure 18-3)

1. Characteristics

Epiphyseal separation occurs at the elbow and is more common in infants and toddlers. Supracondylar fracture of the elbow is a <u>hyperextension</u> injury common in children 3 to 8 years of age. Fracture may be combined with dislocation of the elbow with the risk of neurovascular injury (Figure 18-3).

2. Management

The arm should be splinted in slight flexion. Neurovascular status should be assessed carefully. In most cases of vascular compromise, the treatment is reduction.

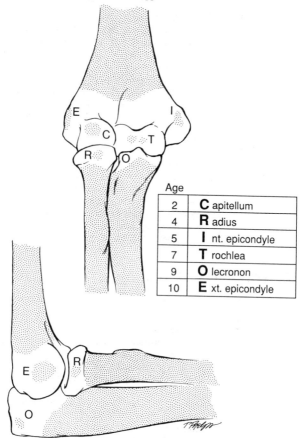

Age	
2	**C** apitellum
4	**R** adius
5	**I** nt. epicondyle
7	**T** rochlea
9	**O** lecronon
10	**E** xt. epicondyle

Figure 18-3. Anterior-posterior and lateral view of the child's elbow demonstrating sequence of ossification by age: Capitellum, Radius, Internal Epicondyle, Olecranon, External Epicondyle.

B. **Pelvic and Femur Fractures**

1.   Characteristics
     These represent the fractures most likely to be associated with significant blood loss. Torn blood vessels with or without fractured cancellous bone may account for large blood losses with pelvic fractures (10-15% of blood volume). Anterior-posterior compression injuries are most likely to produce urologic injury (5-15% of pelvic fractures).

2.   Signs of associated urologic injury include:
     blood at meatus, inability to pass urine, local trauma to perineum, and a high prostate.

3.   Management of pelvic fracture (+ urologic injury)
     a.   Obtain a retrograde urethrogram (+/- cystogram)
     b.   No urethral catheterization in suspicious cases without prior contrast studies.

4.   Management of femur fracture
     Use a Hare splint for femur fractures which immobilizes the extremity up to the pelvis and applies slight traction. Neurovascular status should be checked. (See *Chapter 10* for nerve block.)

C.   Spine Fractures

1.   Pediatric differences
     The spine is normally more mobile in children such that up to 3 mm pseudosubluxation at the 2nd

and 3rd cervical vertebrae may be a normal variant. The ossification sequence of the cervical spine varies which makes radiographic interpretation of fractures more difficult. The normal pediatric cervical spine is diagrammed in Figure 18-4.

2. Management
Suspected cervical spine injuries are managed according to an emergency algorithm (Figure 18-5).

a. Radiographic Interpretation
The thoracolumbar spine should be x-rayed if the physician is unable to establish lack of spine tenderness and a normal neurologic exam. Rarely, children may have SCIWORA - Spinal Cord Injury Without Radiographic Abnormality - so that spine injury may have to be diagnosed on clinical grounds alone. Thus the spine should be handled with reasonable care in all unresponsive children following severe trauma, even if x-rays are normal.

b. Steroids
A recent study (Bracken, N Engl J Med 322: 20, 1990) has suggested that neurologic recovery after acute spinal cord injury is improved by prompt (within 8 hrs) administration of:

Methylprednisolone 30 mg/kg IV (loading dose)

followed by

Methylprednisolone 5.4 mg/kg/hr IV (infusion).

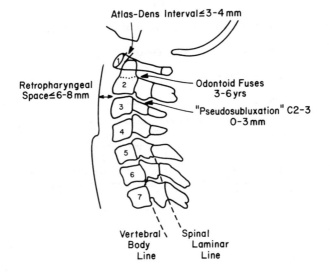

Figure 18-4. Features of normal pediatric cervical spine.

Unconscious Patient	Major Facial and Head Trauma	Neck Tenderness or Neurologic Deficit

↘   ↓   ↙

Treat as Cervical Spine Fracture
↓

No neck motion during airway management

↓

Immobilize on backboard with:
sandbags and tape or cervical collar

↓

Brief neuro exam (strength and sensation in extremities)

↓

Consult orthopedist and neurosurgeon

↓

Radiographic studies

↓

Resting lateral x-ray of cervical spine

↓

If lateral view abnormal:	For neck tenderness or questionable neck stability:
↓	↓
Anterior-posterior and open-mouth x-ray or CT scan	Active flexion/extension views under patient's own power

↓

Use MRI of the spine for certain neuro deficits

Figure 18-5. Management algorithm for suspected cervical spine injury.

D. Compartment Syndrome (CS)

1. Mechanism of injury

   CS develops because of increased compartment contents and a limiting fascial envelope. Increased contents include hemorrhage and cellular swelling from ischemia or blunt trauma. When compartment pressure is greater than capillary perfusion pressure (30-45 mmHg), ischemia further aggravates compartment swelling.

2. Evaluation

   Clinical signs of CS described as the "5 P's":

   a. Pain is out of proportion to the expected. The most sensitive finding in the physical exam is exquisite pain in passive stretch of the involved muscles (Figure 18-6).

   b. Paresthesia arises from sensory nerves coursing through compartment.

   c. Pallor occurs in the distal part of the extremity with poor capillary refill (> 3 seconds).

   d. Pulselessness in the distal extremity is a very late sign.

   e. Paralysis is also a late sign; early weakness should be sought instead.

   CS is suspected even if only <u>one</u> of the findings is present. Assessment relies on the measurement of compartment pressure with sterile needle, syringe, stopcock and manometer (Whitesides method), or with a commercially available device (Figure 18-7). Critical pressure depends on mean blood pressure, but in general treatment is initiated when compartment pressure is > 30-45 mmHg.

3. Outcome

   The duration of increased compartment pressure determines outcome:

   a. < 6 hrs → Good outcome in 95% of patients after fasciotomy.

   b. > 12 hrs → Good outcome in only 6% of patients after fasciotomy.

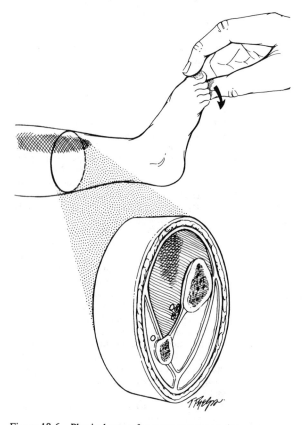

Figure 18-6. Physical exam for compartment syndrome.
In the anterior compartment of the leg, plantar flexion of the toes stretches the toe extensors (shaded) causing pain, yet does not cause movement of any long bone fractures which may be present.

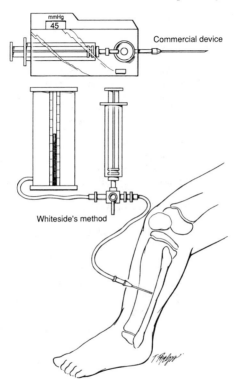

Figure 18-7. Whiteside's method for measurement of compartment pressure. The sterile needle, inserted into the compartment, is attached to fluid-filled tubing, a 3-way stopcock, and a manometer. A 30 ml, air-filled syringe is attached to the stopcock which is open to the syringe and the tubing. Air is injected from the syringe until a small air bubble in the tubing is displaced toward the needle and the corresponding manometer pressure is recorded. Commercial devices measure compartment pressure automatically.

IV. PRACTICAL POINTS

A. Open Fractures

1. Cultures should be obtained from the wound on presentation in the emergency room.
2. Antibiotic therapy: Include antistaphycoccal coverage (e.g, a cephalosporin).
3. For severely contaminated, massive crush - or farm injuries: Add gentamicin and penicillin for Gram negative rod and streptococcal coverage.
4. Early operative debridement and irrigation is indicated in most cases, within 6 hours of injury.
5. Tetanus prophylaxis (See Table 19-1).

B. Reimplantation of Amputated Extremity

1. Virtually never attempted for leg amputation, unless very "clean."
2. Consider in <u>clean</u> hand/arm cases.
3. Do not pack the amputated extremity directly on ice, rather it should be protected in a plastic bag, then cooled.
4. Call reimplant center in advance.

Chapter 19
SOFT TISSUE INJURIES

I. OVERVIEW

A. Definition
Soft tissue injuries include all bodily trauma except head and nervous system, solid organs, body cavities, and long bones. These injuries also include the familiar "lumps and bumps of childhood" which are rarely life-threatening, but are very threatening to child and family because the child is awake and scared during the evaluation and treatment.

B. Priorities
1. Primary Survey
   Soft tissue injury is generally obvious to the clinician during the primary survey. The primary survey should exclude skeletal or skull fractures associated with soft tissue trauma and penetration into body cavities.
2. Hemostasis
3. Tetanus prophylaxis (Tables 19-1, 19-2)
4. Wound irrigation and debridement
5. Sedation and Analgesia
   Sedation may be necessary, setting the stage for a more careful controlled evaluation of extensive soft tissue injury, <u>after</u> primary survey is accomplished. Local anesthetics should be introduced into lacerations which will require meticulous suturing for good cosmetic results. (See *Chapter 10*.)

II. OPEN FRACTURES (See *Chapter 18*)

A. Characteristics
Frequently, long bone fractures are associated with overlying soft tissue injuries. This increases the possibility of hemorrhage and infection.

    B.   **Management**
        1.   Hemorrhage is controlled with direct pressure.
        2.   The open wound is covered with a sterile dressing.
        3.   The fractured extremity is immobilized with a rigid posterior splint.
        4.   Definitive management takes place in the operating room under anesthesia.

III. CLOSED DISPLACED FRACTURES

    A.   **Characteristics**
    Displaced fractures may be associated with extensive soft tissue injuries as a result of the movement of bone fragments within the surrounding tissues. This may result in disruption of major vascular structures.

    B.   **Management**
        1.   Control of major hemorrhage.
        2.   Immediate immobilization to avoid blood loss and hematoma formation.
        3.   Continuous monitoring of pulse, capillary refill and sensation to insure neurovascular integrity of distal extremity and detect a compartment syndrome early. (See *Chapter 18*)
        4.   Early consultation with an orthopedic surgeon.

IV. CONTUSIONS

    A.   **Characteristics**
    Contusions may be relatively superficial, like bruises, or they may be much deeper when associated with intramuscular hemorrhage and bleeding into joint spaces. Rarely, a closed compartment syndrome may be associated with such deep contusions.

B. **Management**
   1.   Usually self limiting.
   2.   Early immobilization will enhance resolution.
   3.   Large deep seated hematomas require drainage if signs of compartment syndrome are present.

V. LACERATIONS

Lacerations or open skin wounds require urgent evaluation and treatment because delay allows for bacterial growth with eventual complications of local and systemic infection.

A. **Classification**
   1.   Dirty Wound
        The dirty wound is grossly contaminated by body excreta or by contaminants from the environment.
   2.   Clean Wound
        A clean wound is not contaminated nor does it contain foreign material.
   3.   Mangled Wound
        The mangled laceration, such as a dog bite, has a crushing component with distortion of tissues other than the simple transection of the skin and underlying fatty tissue. They should probably be seen by a plastic surgeon because excision of some of the damaged tissue may be necessary.
   4.   Sharp Wound
        Tissues are simply transected but not distorted.
   5.   Facial vs. Extremity Wounds
        The location of the laceration is critical because a facial laceration has greater cosmetic distortion and potential for more dangerous infection than does one over the body or extremities. Extremity lacerations carry with them the potential for deep penetration and involvement of tendons or nerves.

B. Management

1. Irrigation

   Prompt, gentle irrigation and cleansing with sterile saline or H_2O diminishes the threat of infection.

2. Debridement

   In mangled lacerations, the devitalized tissue requires excision/debridement. Consider plastic surgical consultation. (Figure 19-1)

3. Suturing

   Most lacerations ultimately require some type of suturing for approximation of tissues (Figure 19-2). Absorbable suture material (e.g., Vicryl) is used for subcutaneous sutures and removable, monofilament sutures (e.g., Nylon) for superficial suturing. Alternative closure techniques are possible in special situations (Figure 19-3).

4. Primary Closure

   Clean wounds may be closed primarily.

   Properly irrigated and debrided dirty wounds may be closed primarily within 6 hours of the time of injury.

5. Secondary Closure

   If the wound is >6 hours old, it is best treated openly with antibiotics and wet/dry sterile saline compresses and then repaired secondarily.

6. Antibiotic Coverage

   For clean wounds of the body and extremities prophylactic antibiotics are rarely indicated. For facial lacerations and penetrating injuries to the hands and feet, consider prophylactic antibiotics for 48-72 hours.

7. Tetanus prophylaxis (Tables 19-1, 19-2)

8. Outcome

   A sharp, clean wound will heal with minimal scarring, while the improperly treated mangled wound may require future plastic reconstruction.

TABLE 19-1. Tetanus Prophylaxis

Tetanus Immunization Status	Interval Since Last Dose	Type of Prophylaxis	
		Clean Wounds	Dirty Wounds
≤3 DPT or uncertain		*Td O.5 ml IM	Td 0.5 ml & **TIG 250 units IM
>3 DPT	<5 yrs	None	None
	5-10 yrs	None	Td 0.5 ml IM
	>10 yrs	Td 0.5 ml IM	Td 0.5 ml IM

* Tetanus Toxoid   ** Tetanus Immune Globulin

TABLE 19-2. Assessment of Wounds for Tetanus Prophylaxis

Clinical Features	Tetanus-Prone Wound	Nontetanus-Prone Wound
Age of wound	> 6 hours	≤ 6 hours
Configuration	Stellate wound, avulsion, abrasion	Linear wound
Depth	> 1 cm	≤1 cm
Mechanism of injury	Missile, crush, burn, frostbite	Sharp surface (glass, knife)
Signs of infection	Present	Absent
Devitalized tissue	Present	Absent
Contamination	Present	Absent

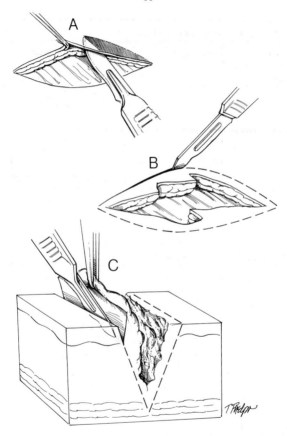

Figure 19-1. Undermining the skin edges with scalpel or scissors will relieve tension on closure (A). Minimal debridement of devitalized edges and imbedded foreign material will improve the cosmetic result (B,C). Gentle handling of tissue prevents further injury.

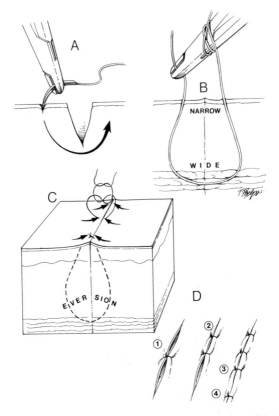

Figure 19-2.   Passing the needle in an arc (A) to obtain a slightly wider base than top (B) will result in the desired slight eversion of the wound edges (C). Placement of simple interrupted sutures usually provides the precise alignment necessary for best appearance of the wound.   Suture placement splitting the difference in the wound's length aids in obtaining the best apposition (D).

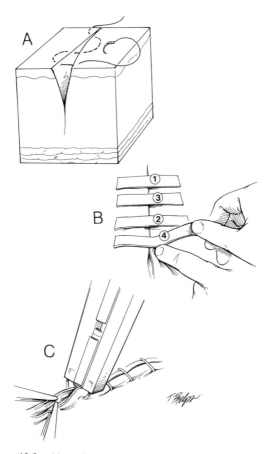

Figure 19-3. Alternatives to interrupted suture placement include a running subcuticular technique (A), sterile adhesive strip application (B), skin staple placement (C).

VI. ABRASIONS

A. Management of Simple Abrasions

1. Topical cleansing with soap and water and a dry sterile dressing.
2. Topical antibiotic (e.g., Bacitracin) to prevent adherence of the dressing.

B. Management of Deeper Abrasions

1. Debridement and brushing to remove the particles (e.g., gravel). This may require general anesthesia.
2. Failure to remove particulate foreign bodies may result in a "road rash" or "abrasion tatoo" for months or years.
3. Tetanus prophylaxis (Tables 19-1 and 19-2)

VII. OUTCOME OF SOFT TISSUE INJURIES

The eventual outcome of soft tissue injuries is usually excellent in children because their tissues are young and growing which is a basic setting for good healing. In addition, children rarely have systemic diseases or skin infections which would interfere with healing.

Chapter 20
BURNS

I. OVERVIEW

Thermal injuries involve one million children each year. Ten percent require hospitalization each year. Permanent disability remains the major complication. Eighty to ninety percent of thermal injuries occur in the home and they are preventable. Scald injury is the most common burn in children under three years, involving boys twice as often as girls. Flame burns involve both sexes equally and are most common over the age of three years.

II. PATHOPHYSIOLOGY

A. Scald Injuries
1. Full thickness injury in adults
   a. Exposure to 70°C (158°F) burns in less than one second
   b. Exposure to 52°C (125°F) burns in 120 seconds
2. Because of their thin skin, full thickness injuries occur in less time in children.

B. Depth of Burn
1. First degree - erythema, pain, absence of blisters
2. Second degree - partial thickness, erythema, swelling, blisters, hypersensitive skin, weeping
3. Third degree - full thickness, pale or leathery, dry, edematous, insensitive skin

C. Fluid Shifts
1. Partial - and full thickness injuries result in increased capillary permeability and sequestration of large quantities of fluid.
2. Larger surface area causes children to lose more fluid and body heat than adults.

D. Inhalation Injuries
1. Injuries are due to products of incomplete combustion, toxic fumes and/or direct thermal injury.
2. Manifestations may not be apparent for 24 hours.

III. IMMEDIATE LIFE-SAVING MEASURES
(Figure 20-1)

A. Airway
1. Indications for endotracheal intubation
   a. Facial burns
   b. Singed eyebrows and nasal hairs
   c. Carbon deposits and inflammatory changes of the pharynx
   d. Carbonaceous sputum
   e. Stridor or hoarseness
   f. Confinement in a burning environment
   g. Altered level of consciousness
   h. Restrictive ventilation secondary to circumferential full thickness injury of the chest.
2. The physicians must be aware of early signs of injury; delay may make intubation very difficult.

B. Stop the Burning Process
All clothing must be removed to prevent further burn injury and to allow complete assessment.

C. Intravenous Access
1. Required when >15% burn surface area.
2. Unburned area preferred for access.
3. If unable to obtain IV access, intraosseous infusion should be used.
4. Preferred fluid: Lactated Ringer's - 20 ml/kg/hr
5. Urine output goal: 1-2 ml/kg/hr
6. Shock: Lactated Ringer's I.V. bolus 20 ml/kg, repeat twice if necessary.

MANAGEMENT OF LIFE THREATENING BURNS

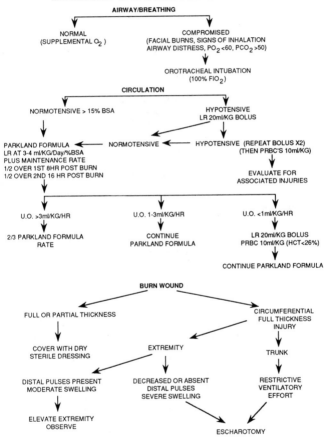

Figure 20-1. Primary Survey of Life-Threatening Burns.
LR - Lactated Ringer's solution. U.O. - urine output.

IV. ASSESSING THE BURN INJURY

A. History

1. When, where and how burn injury occurred

2. Past medical history

   a. Pre-existing medical problems
   b. Tetanus immunizations
      (Tables 19-1 and 19-2)
   c. Allergies
   d. Intercurrent infections

3. Careful history may determine child abuse or other traumatic injuries.

B. Estimating Severity

1. Determination of severity is important in fluid and wound management as well as predicting morbidity and mortality.

2. Depth of injury determined as summarized in II.B.

3. Burn surface area (BSA)
   The modified Lund and Browder Chart is used to determine % burn surface area (Figure 20-2) in children.

4. Chemical and electrical injuries
   Burn wound severity is under estimated in chemical and electrical injuries because often the underlying soft tissue injury is not evident.

Burn Estimate Age vs Area

Area	Birth 1yr.	1-4 yr.	5-9 yr.	10-14 yr.	15 yr.	2°	3°	Total
Head	19	17	13	11	9			
Neck	2	2	2	2	2			
Ant. Trunk	13	13	13	13	13			
Post. Trunk	13	13	13	13	13			
R. Buttock	2 1/2	2 1/2	2 1/2	2 1/2	2 1/2			
L. Buttock	2 1/2	2 1/2	2 1/2	2 1/2	2 1/2			
Genitalia	1	1	1	1	1			
R.U. Arm	4	4	4	4	4			
L.U. Arm	4	4	4	4	4			
R.L. Arm	3	3	3	3	3			
L.L. Arm	3	3	3	3	3			
R. Hand	2 1/2	2 1/2	2 1/2	2 1/2	2 1/2			
L. Hand	2 1/2	2 1/2	2 1/2	2 1/2	2 1/2			
R. Thigh	5 1/2	6 1/2	8	8 1/2	9			
L. Thigh	5 1/2	6 1/2	8	8 1/2	9			
R. Leg	5	5	5 1/2	6	6 1/2			
L. Leg	5	5	5 1/2	6	6 1/2			
R. Foot	3 1/2	3 1/2	3 1/2	3 1/2	3 1/2			
L. Foot	3 1/2	3 1/2	3 1/2	3 1/2	3 1/2			
					Total			

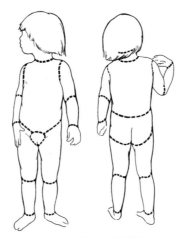

Figure 20-2. Burn surface area estimate (BSA) by area. Shade areas of figure to correspond with patient's burn areas. Determine burn estimate by age by adding the percentages using the chart.

V. SECONDARY SURVEY (Figure 20-3)

A. Airway

1. Serial re-evaluation of the patient is necessary throughout the stabilization period.
2. Treatment of carbon monoxide exposure is diagrammed in Figure 20-4.

B. Rapid Assessment of Associated Injuries

1. Neurologic deficit
   a. Glasgow Coma Scale (Table 15-1)
   b. Focal findings
2. Thoraco-abdominal injuries (*Chapter 16 and 17*)
   a. Tension pneumothorax
   b. Flail chest, pulmonary contusion
   c. Solid organ injury with hemorrhage
3. Orthopedic injuries
   a. Long bone or pelvic injuries
   b. Spinal injury
   c. Compartment syndrome

C. Assessment of Fluid Resuscitation

1. Parkland formula
   When BSA >15%, IV fluid replacement is guided by the Parkland formula: Lactated Ringer's 3-4 ml/kg/day/%BSA plus maintenance fluids *(Chapter 5)*. Give 1/2 over the first 8 hours and the remainder over the next 16 hours.
2. Urine output
   Urine output is measured to determine adequacy of IV fluid replacement.
3. Foley catheter for >30% BSA
4. CVP or Swan-Ganz catheter for >50% BSA

BURN WOUND MANAGEMENT

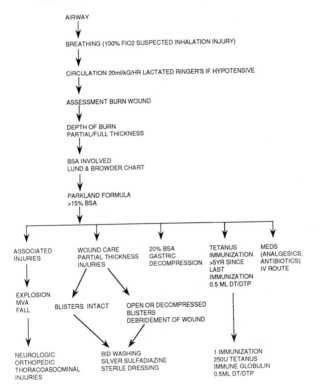

Figure 20-3. Management of the burn patient.

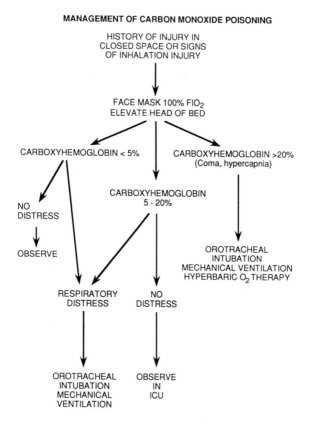

Figure 20-4. Management of carbon monoxide poisoning.

D. Burn Wound Management

1. Wound Care -
   Aseptic technique is mandatory.

   a. Blisters are left intact.
   b. Open blisters and necrotic tissue are debrided.
   c. Cover wounds with dry sterile linen.
   d. Escharotomy is indicated for circumferential full thickness injury to chest or extremities.

2. Laboratory Studies

   a. CBC
   b. Electrolytes
   c. Chemistry profile
   d. Type and crossmatch
   e. Arterial blood gas, carboxyhemoglobin

3. Radiographs

   a. Chest
   b. Evaluation of associated injuries

4. Gastric decompression

   a. Ileus common if > 20% BSA
   b. Nasogastric tube may be used for feedings once intestinal function has returned.

5. Medication

   a. No antibiotic prophylaxis
   b. Intravenous route for analgesia and sedation
   c. Evaluate hypoxia and hypovolemia prior to treatment of restless or anxious child.

VI. ELECTRICAL BURNS (Figure 20-5)

A. Overview

Electrical burns are more serious than their external appearance. Electrical current damages muscle, nerve, and blood vessels. Immediate management: as outlined for other types of burns under III.A.B.C.

B. Secondary Assessment

1. Intracranial or spinal injuries
2. Thoracic and abdominal injuries
3. Compartment syndrome and long bone fractures
4. Entrance and exit wound sites

C. Rhabdomyolysis - Myoglobinuria

1. I.V. fluid administered at rate to maintain urine output of 3-5 ml/kg/hr

2. Mannitol 500 mg/kg bolus

3. Alkalinization of urine - sodium bicarbonate I.V. (1-2 mEq/kg)

4. Monitor for life-threatening hyperkalemia.

D. Injury to Corner of Mouth

1. Frequent injury in toddler
2. Topical antibiotic therapy
3. Allow wound demarcation prior to surgical debridement
4. Early involvement of plastic surgeon

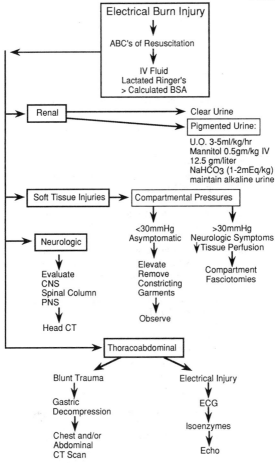

Figure 20-5. Management of electrical burn.

VII. GUIDELINES FOR TRIAGE AND DISPOSITION (Table 20-1)

A. Overview

Admit child when etiology and/or extent in question. Develop transfer protocols to facilitate early, safe transport of the pediatric patient.

B. Outpatient Management

1. Cleanse wound with sterile saline or mild antibacterial solution.

2. Blisters should be left intact. Open or leaking blisters are debrided.

3. For partial thickness burns on the extremities silver sulfadiazine is applied BID and the wound is covered with an occlusive dressing (*Chapter 19*).

4. Partial thickness facial burns: Apply Bacitracin ointment BID (Table 20-2).

5. Physician observation every 48 hours for:
   a. Wound depth and extent.
   b. Wound infection.

6. Oral hydration.

7. Acetaminophen or codeine for pain (*Chapter 10*).

8. Tetanus immunization.

9. Partial thickness burns should epithelialize in 14 - 21 days.

TABLE 20-1. Triage Criteria for Thermal Injuries

- **Outpatient Management**

  Partial thickness burn <10% BSA
  Full thickness burn <2% BSA

- **Inpatient Management/Primary care hospital**

  Partial thickness burn 10-20% BSA
  Full-thickness burn 2-10% BSA
  Partial thickness burn to face, perineum, hands or feet
  Questionable burn wound depth or extent
  Inadequate family support
  Suspected abuse

- **Burn Center**

  Partial thickness burn >20% BSA
  Full-thickness burn >10% BSA
  Full-thickness burn to face, perineum, hands or feet
  Respiratory tract injury
  Associated major trauma
  Significant coexisting illness
  Chemical or electrical burns

TABLE 20-2. Topical Antibacterial Agents

AGENT	ACTION	SIDE EFFECTS	WOUND THERAPY
Bacitracin ointment	limited activity/poor eschar penetration	Conjunctivitis; development of resistant organisms	Apply to small areas of partial thickness burns of face twice daily
Silver Sulfadiazine	Broad activity; painless; fair penetration of eschar	Sulfa sensitivity (rash); transient leukopenia	Apply daily; cover extremities with light dressing; leave face and trunk open
Mafenide	Excellent broad spectrum coverage; penetrates eschar rapidly	Painful; sulfa sensitivity; carbonic anhydrase inhibition (acidosis)	Apply thin layer daily; cover extremities with light dressing; leave face and trunk open
Aqueous silver nitrate solution	Excellent broad spectrum coverage; poor eschar penetration	Hypochloremic alkalosis; stains tissues; hypothermia (evaporation)	Apply twice daily; cover with gauze dressing

C. Burn Center Management

1. Specialists of burn center provide for physical, psychological and social needs of the pediatric patient.

2. Criteria for transfer (Table 20-1).

3. Prior to transfer, the injured child must be fully assessed and resuscitated. During transfer adequate ventilation, hemodynamic stability and normothermia are ensured (Table 20-3).

4. All pertinent information sent with the patient.

TABLE 20-3. Transport of the Burn Patient

- **Secure Airway**
  Orotracheal intubation if signs of injury

- **Fluid Resuscitation**
  Secure venous access
  Initiate fluid therapy >15% BSA

- **Thermal Control**
  Cover wounds dry clean or sterile linen
  Blankets
  Heating devices

- **Resuscitation Flow Sheet**
  Fluids
  Urinary output
  Vital signs
  Laboratory results/X-rays

Chapter 21
ORGANIZATION OF EQUIPMENT

I. INTRODUCTION

Selection and Organization of Equipment

1. The selection of emergency equipment and space should reflect the patient populations being served, the skills of the health care personnel, and the additional resources available to supplement emergency care.

2. The organization of space to provide emergency care should be accessible to patients and personnel, should provide privacy from other patient care areas, and should be spacious enough to enable the delivery of safe, unobstructed care.

3. Specific standards are set by the Joint Commission on Accreditation of Healthcare Organizations (JCAHO) for facility design and equipment for the following areas: (1) Emergency Services, (2) Hospital-Sponsored Ambulatory Care Services, and (3) Special Care Units.

II. THE EMERGENCY CRASH CART

A. Emergency Cart Supplies

The cart contents should include sufficient amounts and types of equipment necessary for initial resuscitation. The equipment should be organized in a logical format to allow prompt access of the correct equipment needed in the prescribed, preferred order.

a. Supply variety
One cart can contain supplies for use in all pediatric patients (infants to adolescents).

b. Overall storage design
The design of the cart should allow organized space for equipment of different sizes and shapes. A useful cart is a multi-drawered tool type chest with three drawers and an open-spaced compartment on the bottom of the cart (Figure 21-1).

c. Cart security
The cart should have the capabilities of being locked with routine checking of the integrity of the cart by assigned personnel. If an unlocked cart is used, its contents should be checked at least every shift or after each use by an appropriately assigned person.

d. Equipment distribution
The cart contents should be organized in a manner that facilitates use by all personnel. The top drawer is designated for equipment used for airway management (Figure 21-1). The second drawer contains equipment used for respiratory care and blood drawing (Figure 21-2). The third drawer is designated for equipment used for IV insertion (Figure 21-3). The bottom shelf contains equipment that is large in size (Figure 21-4). A backboard can be placed on the back of the emergency cart (Table 21-1).

TABLE 21-1. Pediatric Emergency Equipment

Drawer 1 (Airway Supplies)
    Laryngoscope handles, blades, bulbs, and batteries
    Endotracheal tubes one each -
        uncuffed 2.5 - 5.5, cuffed 6,7,8
    Stylettes (1 short, 1 long)
    Airways - sizes 00,0,1,2,3,4,5
    Nasal airways - sizes 12 to 32 French
    Oxygen tubing and flowmeter
    Miscellaneous supplies - tape, cotton tip applicators,
        Benzoin, protective eyeware, ECG paper,
                arrest form (if available)
Drawer 2 (Respiratory Care and Blood Drawing)
    Suction catheters - sizes 6,8,10,14,18;
    Yankauer suction catheter
    Pulse oximeter sensors - sizes pediatric and adult
    2 blood gas kits
    Miscellaneous supplies -
        iodine tincture, alcohol wipes, sterile gloves,
        various sized syringes and butterfly needles,
        tourniquets, blood tubes, thoracentesis needle
Drawer 3 (IV insertion)
    Venous catheters - sizes 16,18,20,22,24 gauge
    Intraosseous needle - sizes 16,18
    IV infusion sets, solutions, tubing, stopcocks
    Armboards, gauze, tape, alcohol wipes, gloves
    Miscellaneous supplies -
        gastric tubes, irrigating solution and syringe
Bottom Shelf (oversized equipment)
    Resuscitation bag - pediatric and adult
        with masks - Adult 4,5, pediatric 0,1,3
    Pediatric cutdown set
    Pediatric tracheostomy set with trach tubes
    Oxygen tank and wrench

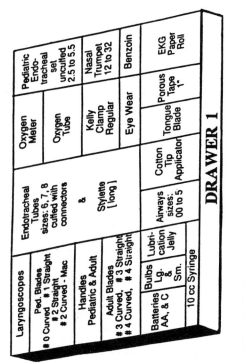

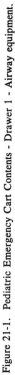

Figure 21-1. Pediatric Emergency Cart Contents - Drawer 1 - Airway equipment.

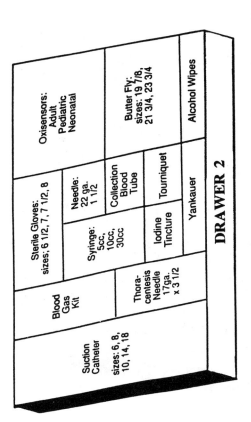

DRAWER 2

Suction Catheter sizes: 6, 8, 10, 14, 18

Blood Gas Kit

Thoracentesis Needle 17ga. x 3 1/2

Sterile Gloves: sizes; 6 1/2, 7, 7 1/2, 8

Needle: 22 ga. 1 1/2

Syringe: 5cc, 10cc, 30cc

Collection Blood Tube

Iodine Tincture

Tourniquet

Oxisensors: Adult Pediatric Neonatal

Butter Fly: sizes: 19 7/8, 21 3/4, 23 3/4

Yankauer

Alcohol Wipes

Figure 21-2. Pediatric Emergency Cart Contents - Drawer 2 - Respiratory care and blood drawing.

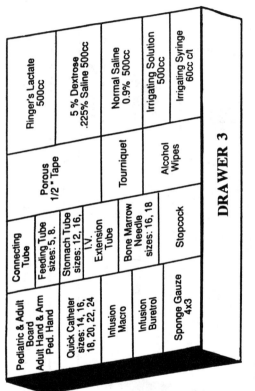

Figure 21-3. Pediatric Emergency Cart Contents - Drawer 3 - Equipment for IV insertion.

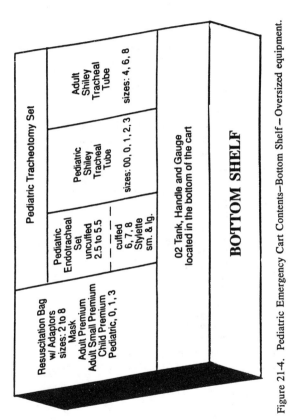

Figure 21-4. Pediatric Emergency Cart Contents—Bottom Shelf—Oversized equipment.

B. Emergency Drugs

A locked box containing pediatric resuscitation and emergency drugs can be placed on top of the crash cart. The integrity of this box should be checked and maintained by appropriately assigned personnel. The drug box will contain drugs and a variety of sizes of syringes and needles (Table 21-2).

TABLE 21-2. Pediatric Emergency Drug Box Contents

Sodium Bicarbonate
Epinephrine
Atropine
Calcium Chloride, Calcium gluconate
Lidocaine
Naloxone
Dextrose 25%
Aminophylline
Bretylium
Diphenhydramine
Dopamine
Glucagon
Hydrocortisone
Isoproterenol
Phenobarbital
Phenytoin
Propranolol

III. OFFICE SUPPLIES

Equipment and Medications

1. The equipment and drugs necessary to treat emergencies of Airway, Breathing and Circulation are listed in Tables 21-3 and 21-4. This equipment should provide the office staff with the ability to assess and stabilize patients before transfer to a designated facility by trained emergency medical systems personnel.

2. The choices of equipment are based on the type and number of patients seen, space in the facility, and cost of equipment. One designated area is used for all emergencies.

3. The staff should be regularly trained in the use and location of this equipment.

TABLE 21-3. Office Equipment

Airway/ Breathing	Portable Oxygen tank
	Suction machine
	O_2 face mask and nasal prongs (Table 2-2)
	Bag-valve - mask device with reservoir
	Plastic masks - sizes 0,1,2,3,4
	Oral airways - sizes 00,0,1,2,3,4,5
	Nasal airways - one of each size 12-32
	Laryngoscope blades, handles, tubes
	Suction catheters - sizes 6,8,10,14
Circulation	Arrest board
	Intravenous fluid administration supplies catheters, butterfly needles, tubing, fluids,
	Intraosseous needles - sizes 16,18
	Sphygmomanometer with various sized cuffs
Miscellaneous Supplies	Gastric tubes - sizes 5,8,12,14 F
	Activated charcoal
	Trauma supplies including dressings and bandages

TABLE 21-4. Medications for Office Use

> Epinephrine (1:10,000)
> Sodium Bicarbonate
> Atropine
> Calcium chloride
> Dextrose
> Aminophylline
> Phenytoin (Dilantin)
> Phenobarbital
> Diazepam (Valium) injectable
> Naloxone
> Ipecac

IV. AMBULANCE TRANSPORT

Selection of Equipment

1. Selection of equipment for use in ambulances should follow the specific standards legislated by existing municipal, county or state authorities.

2. The equipment must meet the needs of patients of all ages and sizes patients. This is best organized by equipment type rather than by age.

3. Specific equipment necessary to care for pediatric patients includes airway management supplies, venous access supplies, monitoring supplies including ECG and pulse oximetry, pediatric MAST and traction supplies (Table 21-5).

TABLE 21-5.   Ambulance Equipment for the Pediatric Patient

Airway management supplies
> Pediatric oxygen delivery systems
>> face mask, nasal cannulas - sizes infant, child
> Oropharyngeal airways - sizes 00,0,1,2,3,4
> Hand operated infant bag resuscitator unit
>> oxygen inlet, reservoir tube, pop-off valve, masks
> Suction catheters - sizes 6,8,10,14

Venous access supplies
> IV catheters - 20,22,24 gauge
> IV administration sets - micro infusion set

Monitoring supplies
> Blood pressure cuffs - sizes infant and child
> ECG cable with pediatric monitoring electrodes
> Pulse oximetry sensors
> Pediatric stethoscope

Other
> Pediatric stiffneck collar
> Pediatric HARE (traction) splint, splint board
> Pediatric MAST

V.   HELICOPTER TRANSPORT

Selection of Equipment

1. The selection of equipment for use in air medical transport should adhere to the regulations set by state regulatory boards and/or the Federal Aviation Administration. The specific equipment on a given helicopter is determined by the mission of the transporting service, types of patients transported and the accompanying personnel.

2. Because of the space constraints, it is best to separate and organize specific equipment by age, i.e., pediatric equipment separated from adult equipment. Organization of equipment in a carrying bag would include supplies necessary for airway management, venous access, and monitoring (Table 21-6).

TABLE 21-6. Equipment for Pediatric Flight Bag

Airway management supplies
>   Oxygen delivery systems -
>   face masks, nasal cannulas
>   Pediatric Ambu bag with masks
>   Intubation kit
>   Endotracheal tubes 2.5,3,4,5,6
>   Laryngoscope handle with blade sizes
>   0,1,2 straight, 2 curved
>   Tracheostomy tubes - sizes 00,0,1,2
>   Oral airways - sizes 00,0,1,2,3,4
>   Suction catheters - sizes 6,8,10,14
>   Needle aspiration kit -
>   16 gauge catheter, stopcock, 30cc syringe

Venous access supplies
>   Angiocaths - sizes 18,20,22,24 gauge
>   Butterflies - sizes 21,23,25 gauge
>   Intraosseous needles
>   Buretrols - with microdrips
>   Pediatric sized armboards

Monitoring supplies
>   ECG cable with pediatric monitoring electrodes
>   Blood pressure cuffs - sizes infant and child
>   Pediatric stethoscope

FORMULARY

Body Surface Area Nomogram

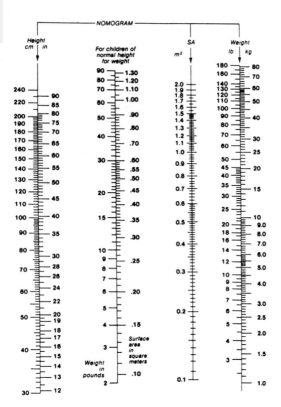

The following is a compendium of drugs used in the advanced pediatric life support. The dosages and indications are intended to be helpful suggestions. Some of these are controversial, however, and should be applied with appropriate caution.

DRUG	SIDE EFFECTS	PHARMACOLOGY
Acetaminophen child: 5-15 mg/kg/dose q4-6h PO, PR; adult: 300-1000 mg q4h; max adult dose: 4000 mg/day	•skin rash •drug fever •hematologic disturbances •contraindicated in G-6-PD deficiency •hepatic necrosis after 200-250 mg/kg	•antipyretic and analgesic, •little anti-inflammatory action
Acetazolamide (Diamox): diuretic and urine alkalinization: 5 mg/kg/dose PO, IV elevated ICP: 25 mg/kg/day PO, IV TID; increased by 25 mg/kg/day up to 100 mg/kg/day; max adult dose 2 gm/day seizures: 8-30 mg/kg/day PO, IV q6-12h	•alkaline urine because of sodium bicarbonate and potassium wasting •systemic metabolic acidosis •drowsiness, paresthesia	•reversible inhibition of carbonic anhydrase •decreases rate of CSF production

Newborns	6 mos	2 yrs	3 yrs	10 yrs	Adults
3 kg	7 kg	12 kg	14 kg	32 kg	70 kg

Acetylcysteine (Mucomyst): acetaminophen toxicity: Oral: Load 140 mg/kg diluted 1:4 in carbonated beverage PO, NG then 70 mg/kg q4h x 17 doses PO, NG; Parenteral: load 150 mg/kg in 200 ml NS over 15 min, then 50 mg/kg in 500 ml NS over 4 hrs, then 100 mg/kg in 1000 ml of NS over 16 hrs	• inhalation: bronchial pain (caution in asthma) • stomatitis • rhinorrhea, bronchorrhea	
Acyclovir Herpes Simplex Virus newborns: 10 mg/kg/dose q8h IV children < 12 years old: 250 mg/M^2/dose q8h IV adults: 5 mg/kg/dose q8h IV Dose given over 1 hr in concentration < 7 mg/ml	• resistance • renal dysfunction • encephalopathy	• activity against HSV I > HSV II • synthetic purine nucleoside analog interacts with viral thymidine kinase
Albuterol (Proventil) Inhalations: 2-90 µg q4-6h Nebulized (5 mg/ml solution): 0.15 mg/kg (max 2 mg); then 0.05 mg/kg q20 min, max 2 mg	• tachycardia • nausea and vomiting • hypertension	• β-2 agonist relaxes bronchial, uterine, and vascular smooth muscle.
Allopurinol (Zyloprim) 10 mg/kg/day ÷ q8h; max 600 mg/day PO	• ↑ theophylline toxicity • rash • hepatomegaly • hematologic abnormalities • nausea and vomiting	• used in hyperuricemic states (gout, antineoplastic therapy) • inhibits xanthine oxidase • alkaline urine ↑ uric acid clearance

Aluminum Hydroxide (Amphogel) Hyperphosphatemia: 50-150 mg/kg/day ÷ q4-6h PO GI bleeding prophylaxis: 1 ml/kg/dose (320 mg/5ml) q1-2h PO	•constipation •hypophosphatemia •hyperaluminemia •delayed gastric emptying •bioavailability affected with hypotension and bradycardia	•↑ mucous secretion •alkalinization of GI contents

Amikacin sulfate (Amikin)
2.5 mg/kg/dose; frequency of dose depends on age and maturity
≤ 7 days: < 28 wks - q24h; 28-34 wks - q18h;
    term - q12h
≥ 7 days: < 28 wks - q18h; 28-34 wks - q12h;
    term - q8h
	•cochlear and vestibular toxicity occurs with high peaks in the absence of low troughs
	•renal cortex toxicity
	•can exacerbate neuromuscular blockade
		•for use in Gram negative infections
		•poor penetration of the CSF

Aminocaproic acid (Amicar) Antifibrinolysis Children IV: 100 mg/kg (or 3 gm/M²) x 1 hr, then 1 gm/M²/h max 18 gm/M²/day PO: 100 mg/kg/dose ÷ q6-8h Adults: 5 gm PO or IV, then 1 gm/h; max 30 gm/day	•hypotension and bradycardia with rapid administration	•antidote for an overdose of fibrinolytic agents •prevents hyperfibrinolysis

Newborns	6 mos	2 yrs	3 yrs	10 yrs	Adults
3 kg	7 kg	12 kg	14 kg	32 kg	70 kg

Aminophylline Load: 3-8 mg/kg over 20 min IV Maintenance: Neonates: 0.2 mg/kg/hr IV 1 month-1 year: 0.2-0.9 mg/kg/hr IV 1-9 years: 0.8-1.1 mg/kg/hr IV adults: 0.5-1.1 mg/kg/hr IV	• tachycardia • nausea and vomiting • seizures	• inhibition of cyclic nucleotide phosphodiesterase • ↑ release of calcium from sarcoplasmic reticulum
Amiodarone (Cordarone) Ventricular tachycardia children: 10 mg/kg/day ÷ q12h PO x 7-10 days, then reduce to 5 mg/kg/day if effective; max dose 15 mg/kg/day for 3-4 weeks adults: Loading dose: 800-1600 mg/day for 1-3 weeks. Maintenance: 600-800 mg/day x 1 month, then 200-400 mg/day	• corneal microdeposits • peripheral neuropathy • thyroid dysfunction • toxic levels >2.5 μg/kg • pulmonary disturbances	• ↑ ventricular fibrillation threshold • slows repolarization and AV conduction • suppresses ventricular tachycardia
Amphotericin B Test: 0.1 mg/kg/dose IV up to max 1 mg/dose. Initial: 0.25 mg/kg/day IV, increase to 1 mg/kg/day over 4 days; max dose 1.5 mg/kg/day	• fever, chills, hypotension, dyspnea, nausea and vomiting • renal toxicity, seizures • thrombocytopenia, anemia • electrolyte disturbances (hypercalciuria and hypokalemia) • pretreatment for chills and rashes: meperidine and/or diphenhydramine and hydrocortisone	• poor penetration of CSF • binds to steroid moiety on fungal cell membrane

Ampicillin ≤ 7 days old: 50-100 mg/kg/day ÷ q12h IV or IM 8-28 days old: 100-200 mg/kg/day ÷ q8h IV or IM children: 50-400 mg/kg/day ÷ q4-6h depending on the infection	• see penicillin • rash at 5-10 days • interstitial nephritis	• see penicillin • higher dose for CNS infection
Amrinone (Inocor) load: 0.75 mg/kg/dose IV, administered over 2-3 min maintenance: 5-10 μg/kg/min IV maximum dose: 10-18 mg/kg/day Do not dilute in glucose containing solutions	• relaxes vascular and tracheal smooth muscle • nausea • thrombocytopenia • ↑ HR and stroke volume • ↓ systemic vascular resistance, left ventricular end diastolic pressure	• positive inotrope • inhibits cyclic nucleotide phosphodiesterase
Aspirin antipyretic: 10-15 mg/kg/dose PO up to 60-80 mg/kg/day antirheumatic: 100 mg/kg/day ÷ q4h	• irreversible platelet dysfunction • acute renal failure • respiratory alkalosis, metabolic acidosis • liver toxicity	• inhibits cyclooxygenase • inhibits the conversion of arachidonic acid to PGG_2
Atracurium muscle relaxant: intubation: 0.6 mg/kg IV	• hypotension	• nondepolarizing relaxant • safe in renal and liver pts

Newborns	6 mos	2 yrs	3 yrs	10 yrs	Adults
3 kg	7 kg	12 kg	14 kg	32 kg	70 kg

Atropine 0.01-0.02 mg/kg IV, IM; min dose 0.15 mg; max dose 1.0 mg (may give via an endotracheal tube)	• ↑ HR • dilated pupils • dry mouth • urinary retention • mental status changes	• muscarinic antagonist, blocks the vagus nerve
Bretylium <u>Life threatening ventricular arrhythmias</u> ≥ 12 years old: 5-10 mg/kg IV q15-30 min; max dose 30 mg/kg Chronic: 5-10 mg/kg IV over 10-30 min q6h	• hypotension • nausea and vomiting • may be useful in unresponsive ventricular fibrillation	• ↑ duration of action potential, refractory period, PR and QT intervals • inhibits release and reuptake of norepinephrine
Calcium Chloride (100 mg/ml) <u>arrest and hyperkalemia</u>: 10-20 mg/kg IV q10min (slowly) Calcium gluconate give 3 times the chloride dose	• subcutaneous injection (infiltrate) can cause slough • bradycardia, arrhythmias	• ↑ cardiac contractility
Captopril (Capoten) <u>neonates</u>: 0.1-0.4 mg/kg/day ÷ q6-24h PO <u>infants</u>: 0.5-1.0 mg/kg/day ÷ q8h PO	• rashes, hypotension • ↓ aldosterone, ↑ renin production • ↓ pulmonary artery pressure, coronary blood flow preserved	• inhibits conversion of angiotensin I to angiotensin II. • useful in the treatment of congestive heart failure
Charcoal, activated 1 gm/kg PO or NG in 70% sorbitol solution	• should not be given with ipecac • secure the airway first if ↓ mental status	• especially useful for drugs with enterohepatic circulation: theophylline, phenobarbital, tricyclics, digoxin, carbamazepine

Chloral Hydrate (Noctec, Aquachloral) 25-75 mg/kg/dose PO or PR, max dose 2 g					• minimal effect on blood pressure or respiration • gastric necrosis • dermatitis • hypotension and apnea with furosemide and anticoagulants	• no analgesic effect • no anxiolysis • produces sleep and may be useful for diagnostic imaging studies
Cimetidine (Tagamet) 5-10 mg/kg q6h PO or IV, max dose 2400 mg/day					• hypersensitivity reactions (rash, dizziness, neutropenia myalgia, diarrhea) • ↓ liver blood flow	• antagonizes histamine-2 receptor • ↓ gastric acidity and volume • ↑ serum theophylline
Clindamycin (Cleocin) 8-40 mg/kg/day ÷ q6h IM, IV, PO max 600 mg/dose IM, 1200 mg/dose IV					• Pseudomembranous colitis • rash, diarrhea, granulocytopenia, neutropenia • potentiates nondepolarizing muscle relaxants	• excellent anaerobic coverage • poor CSF penetration • accumulates in PMN and macrophages
Codeine 0.5-1.2 mg/kg q4-6h PO only We do not recommend parenteral administration.					• see morphine • antitussive • IM administration painful	• see morphine • administer with acetaminophen

Newborns	6 mos	2 yrs	3 yrs	10 yrs	Adults
3 kg	7 kg	12 kg	14 kg	32 kg	70 kg

Dantrolene (Dantrium)
spasticity:
  children: 0.5 mg/kg/dose PO BID then TID after one day, increase by 0.5 mg/kg/day up to 3 mg/kg QID;
  adult: 25 mg PO qD then 25 mg PO BID-QID, increase by 25 increments up to 100 mg PO QID;
  malignant hyperthermia: 1 mg/kg IV repeat PRN up to max of 10 mg/kg then 1-2 mg/kg PO QID
	• hepatotoxicity esp. fulminant hepatitis
	• CNS changes
	• enhances the action of neuromuscular blocker
		• decreases calcium release from the sarcoplasmic reticulum
		• does not alter neuromuscular transmission
		• relaxes muscle contraction associated with upper motor lesions

Desferoxamine (Desferal):
  Iron overdose: 1 gm IM, presence of "vin rose" color to urine indicates significant ingestion.
  Then 500 mg q4h x 2;
  In iron overload with shock: maximal rate 15 mg/kg/hr IV (up to 1 gram in adults) until serum iron level < 300 µg/dl, max 6 gm/day; continue therapy 24 hrs after patient has produced normal color and quantity of urine;
  Chronic overdose in transfusions: 2.0 gm per unit of blood, not given in the same IV as the transfusion
	• pruritus
	• wheals
	• rash
	• anaphylaxis
	• dysuria
	• GI discomfort
	• tachycardia
		• chelates iron
		• for iron levels > 500 µg/dl chelation therapy should commence

Desmopressin (DDAVP):
  Hemophilia A and von Willebrand's disease:
  0.3-0.4 µg/kg/day IV over 15-30 min ÷ q12h
  Diabetes insipidus:
  3 mos-12 yrs: 0.5-3 µg/day intranasal q12-24h
  adults: max 40 µg/day, min dose 2-5 µg
	• hypertension
	• dose must be titrated to lowest effective dose
	• tachyphylaxis
		• constricts smooth muscle
		• analogue of ADH
		• ↑ factor VIII activity in von Willebrand's diseases and hemophilia

Dexamethasone (Decadron):	• see hydrocortisone	• 25 x the anti-inflammatory action of hydrocortisone
ICP elevation: load: 0.5-1.5 mg/kg IV, IM maint: 0.2-0.5 mg/kg/day ÷ q6h		• no sodium retention
Airway edema: 0.25-0.6 mg/kg/dose q6h		• may diminish hearing loss in meningitis
Meningitis: 0.15 mg/kg/dose q6h x 4 days		
Diazepam (Valium):	• ↓ respiration, BP, cardiac output	• anxiolytic, no analgesia
sedation: 0.04-0.2 mg/kg/dose IV q8h;	• not recommended in newborns	• acts at GABA and benzodiazepine receptor
0.2-0.8 mg/kg/day PO ÷ q8h;	• painful on IV injection, poorly absorbed IM	• apnea, especially when used with opioids and as an anti-convulsant
seizures: 0.2-0.5 mg/kg/dose IV q 15-30 min; max 10 mg		
Diazoxide (Hyperstat, Proglycem):	• severe hypotension	• related to the thiazides
Hypertensive Crisis: 1-5 mg/kg IV q30 min up to 300 mg	• renal and hepatic failure	• antidiuretic action as well as arteriolar smooth muscle relaxation
	• ↑ glucose, ↑ uric acid	
	• fluid retention	

| Newborns | 6 mos | 2 yrs | 3 yrs | 10 yrs | Adults |
| 3 kg | 7 kg | 12 kg | 14 kg | 32 kg | 70 kg |

Digoxin: digitalizing dose: 1/2 the dose, then a 1/4 of the dose q8h x 2; IV or IM dose = PO dose in children > 10 years, but is 75% of the PO dose in children < 10 years premature: 20 μg/kg/day PO; full term: 30 μg/kg/day PO; children: 30-40 μg/kg/day PO; maintenance dose: premature: 5 μg/kg/day PO qD; full term: 8-10 μg/kg/day PO qD; children: 8-12 μg/kg/day PO qD	•nausea, diarrhea and vomiting, change in mental status •virtually any dysrhythmia •toxicity is exacerbated by hypokalemia •any drug which can change potassium equilibrium can cause digitalis toxicity (i.e., diuretics, amphotericin B, succinylcholine)	•directly inhibits Na-K ATPase increasing intracellular Ca^{++} and slow inward current •positive inotrope •negative chronotrope •prolonged refractory period in the atria
Diphenhydramine (Benadryl): sedation and antihistamine: 5 mg/kg/d PO, IV, IM ÷ q6h max 50 mg/dose for dystonic reactions in phenothiazine overdose: 1-2 mg/kg IV, max dose 300 mg/day	•dizziness, tinnitus, diplopia •nausea, vomiting, anorexia •anticholinergic effects: dry mouth, urinary retention, tachycardia, changes in mental status, paradoxical excitation in infants	•used for sedation •histamine-1 receptor antagonist •central antitussive •treatment of pruritus •treatment of nausea
Disopyramide (Norpace) Ventricular dysrhythmias: < 1yr: 10-30 mg/kg/day ÷ q6h PO; 1-4 yr: 10-20 mg/kg/day ÷ q6h PO; 4-12 yr: 10-15 mg/kg/day ÷ q6h PO; 12-18 yr: 6-15 mg/kg/day ÷ q6h PO	•cholinergic blockade (10% as potent as Atropine see Atropine) •↓ cardiac output directly and ↑ systemic vascular resistance •hypoglycemia •prolongation of PR interval •apnea	•type I antiarrhythmic slows sinus rate •↓ slope of phase 4 depolarization in Purkinje fibers, prolongs action potential •↑ refractory period •↑ QRS and QT complex

Dobutamine (Dobutrex): 2 µg/kg/min titrate up to effect, max 40 µg/kg/min Preparation for starting dose: $$6 \times \frac{Wt(kg) \times desired\ dose(\mu g/kg/min)}{desired\ rate\ (ml/hr)} = mg\ drug\ per\ 100\ mlNS$$	• β_1 activity increases inotropy • some α_1 agonism at very high doses • lower left ventricular end diastolic pressure • reduction in myocardial oxygen demand while increasing oxygen supply	• no effect on dopaminergic receptors • tachycardia especially when > 20 µg/kg/min • dysrhythmias • contraindicated in hypertrophic subaortic stenosis
Dopamine (Intropin, Depastat): 2-50 µg/kg/min titrated up from the lower dose Preparation: see Dobutamine	• metabolic precursor of norepinephrine • β_1 agonism directly releases norepinephrine • dopaminergic agonism (2-5 µg/kg/min) causes increased renal blood flow • higher rates cause α-1 effects (> 20 µg/kg/min)	• no CNS penetration • tricyclics and MAO inhibitors exaggerate the action
d-Tubo curare: muscle relaxant, intubation: newborn: 0.2 mg/kg IV > 6 wks: 0.6 mg/kg IV	• hypotension • bronchospasm	• histamine release • ganglionic blockade • myocardial depression

Newborns	6 mos	2 yrs	3 yrs	10 yrs	Adults
3 kg	7 kg	12 kg	14 kg	32 kg	70 kg

Edrophonium (Tensilon): test for myasthenia gravis: 0.2 mg/kg/dose IV slowly; range: 0.1-10 mg; Supraventricular tachycardia: 0.1-0.2 mg/kg/dose IV slowly; reversal of neuromuscular blockade: 1 mg/kg IV given with atropine 0.02 mg/kg IV	• see neostigmine • bradycardia	• works faster than any other anti-cholinesterase • see neostigmine
EDTA: Lead poisoning: 1-1.5 gm/M²/day IM ÷ q4-12h for 3-5 days max 75 mg/kg/day IM ÷ BID-TID, IM preferable to IV	• rapid administration causes hypocalcemic seizures • nephrotoxicity • thrombophlebitis • rapid IV administration in patients with cerebral edema may ↑ intracranial pressure • arrhythmia (monitor ECG during IV administration)	• chelates di- and trivalent metals • adequate urine output must be maintained
Ephedrine Hypotension: 0.1-0.2 mg/kg IV		• direct and indirect α and β adrenergic stimulation

	Newborns	6 mos	2 yrs	3 yrs	10 yrs	Adults
	3 kg	7 kg	12 kg	14 kg	32 kg	70 kg

Epinephrine (Adrenalin):
Hypotension: bolus 5-20 µg/kg IV;
infusion 0.05-2 µg/kg/min IV
Resuscitation: 10 µg/kg IV
Preparation: see Dobutamine

- ↑ total leukocye counts, but ↓ eosinophils,
- transient **hyperkalemia** followed by profound **hypokalemia**
- hyperglycemia,
- anxiety, dizziness, palpitations,
- pallor,
- tachyarrhythmias,
- cerebral hemorrhage

- α effects (hypertension) and ß effects (tachycardia)
- activation of adenylate cyclase
- ß₂-agonist relaxes uterine and bronchial smooth muscles
- positive inotrope, chronotrope and dromotrope

Epinephrine (Racemic): Vaponefrin, Micronefrin,
Asthmanefrin Soln 2.25%
Nebulization: 0.05 ml/kg/dose max 0.5 ml diluted in 3 ml
NS q20min x 3

- for use in croup (also post-extubation croup)
- has a risk of rebound airway edema

Erythromycin:
10-20 mg/kg/day ÷ q6h IV, PO

- fever
- eosinophilia, rashes
- hepatitis
- thrombophlebitis
- increases level of theophylline

- macrolide antibiotic
- activity against Gram positive bacteria, mycoplasma, legionella, chlamydia, pertussis
- poor CNS penetration

Esmolol: Tachycardia/Hypertension: load: 500 μg/kg/min x 5 min infusion: 25-100 μg/kg/min titrated to effect	•see propranolol	•β_1 selective (cardioselective) antagonist •see propranolol •$t_{1/2}$ = 9 mins after IV
Fentanyl (Sublimaze): Analgesia/Sedation:1-2 μg/kg/dose IV, up to 100 μg/kg/dose for cardiac anesthesia	•chest wall rigidity due to dopaminergic transmission in the striatum (dose > 5 μg/kg) •see morphine •levels > 1 ng/ml associated with respiratory depression	•specific μ agonist •see morphine •short acting (30 min) •minimal hemodynamic effects
Furosemide (Lasix): Oral: 2 mg/kg/dose q6-8h, max 600 mg/day Parenteral: 1 mg/kg/dose q6-12h IV, IM; max 6 mg/kg single dose	•enhances calcium excretion •↑ excretion of titratable acid and ammonia •enhances renal blood flow •↑ pulmonary venous capacitance by ↓ left ventricular filling pressures •metabolic alkalosis •hyperuricemia •deafness •nephrotoxicity (increased in the presence of cephalosporins and renal-toxic drugs)	•acts on the thick ascending loop of Henle by inhibiting electrolyte reabsorption •mild carbonic anhydrase inhibition •redistributes renal blood flow from medulla to cortex

Gentamicin: 2.5 mg/kg/dose IV, IM; frequency of dose depends on age and maturity: <u>≤ 7 days</u> (< 28 wks: q24h; 28-34 wks: q18h, term q12h) <u>≥ 7 days</u> (< 28 wks: q18h; 28-34 wks: q12h, term q8h) <u>Children</u>: q8h	•cochlear and vestibular toxicity occurs with high peaks in the absence of low troughs •renal cortex toxicity •can exacerbate neuromuscular blockade	•inhibits protein synthesis at the 30s mRNA •for use in Gram negative infections •poor CNS penetration		
Glucagon: <u>For Hypoglycemia</u>: 0.1 mg/kg up to 1 mg IM, SC (1 mg = 1 unit)	•acts only on liver glycogen stores converting them to glucose •increases serum glucose	•stimulates adenylate cyclase •positive inotrope and chronotrope •treats insulin-induced hypoglycemia •relaxes the intestinal tract		
Glycopyrrolate (Robinul): <u>For use with neuromuscular blockade reversal and to</u> <u>decrease airway secretions</u>: 0.01 mg/kg/dose q4-8h IV, IM	•see atropine	•muscarinic blocker with minimal associated tachycardia or mental changes •see atropine		

Newborns	6 mos	2 yrs	3 yrs	10 yrs	Adults
3 kg	7 kg	12 kg	14 kg	32 kg	70 kg

Drug / Dose	Side effects	Mechanism / Notes
Haloperidol (Haldol): Children 3-12 yrs: Sedation: 0.5-1 mg PO Psychosis: 0.05-0.15 mg/kg/day ÷ BID >12 yrs: Sedation: 2-5 mg/dose IM; 1-15 mg PO Psychosis: 2-5 mg/dose q1-8h IM prm; 1-15 mg/day ÷ BID-TID PO	• extrapyramidal side effects • toxic levels 15 ng/ml • sedation • hypotension • lower seizure threshold	• dopaminergic blocker • α_1-blocker
Heparin: (120 international units = 1 mg) bolus: 50-100 units/kg IV maintenance: 10-25 units/kg/hr IV or 100 units/kg/dose q4h IV. Titrate dose to maintain PTT 1.5-2.5 x control values	• lines flushed with heparinized saline have higher fatty acid concentrations interfering with quantification of some drugs (digoxin, propranolol, phenytoin) • chills, fever, anaphylactic shock, hemorrhage, osteoporosis, thrombocytopenia	• reduces serum triglycerides by releasing tissue lipoprotein lipase • heparin accelerates the binding of thrombin to antithrombin III and heparin cofactor II, inactivates factor X • reversal with protamine 1 mg for every 100 units heparin

| Hydralazine (Apresoline):
For Hypertension:
acute: 0.1-0.5 mg/kg/dose IM, IV, q4-6h;
chronic: 0.75-3 mg/kg/day ÷ q6-12h PO | •tachycardia
•increased renin activity
•fluid retention
•increased coronary, renal and cerebral blood flow
•postural hypotension, headache
•lupus-like syndrome in slow acetylators in summer, two months after administration | •directly relaxes arterial vascular smooth muscle |
| Hydrocortisone (Solucortef):
For status Asthmaticus:
loading: 4-8 mg/kg/dose IV; max 250 mg;
maintenance: 8 mg/kg/day ÷ q6h; | •Cushing habitus, psychiatric changes, cataracts, osteoporosis, myopathy, hyperglycemia, peptic ulcers, sodium retention, suppression of adrenal-pituitary axis (up to 9 months after chronic usage)
•abrupt withdrawal: fever, myalgias and arthralgias, pseudotumor cerebri | •physiologic adrenal secretion 20 mg/day
•physiologic level:
16 µg/dl 8 AM,
4 µg/dl 4 PM |

Newborns	6 mos	2 yrs	3 yrs	10 yrs	Adults
3 kg	7 kg	12 kg	14 kg	32 kg	70 kg

Drug / Dose	Side Effects	Action
Indomethacin (Indocin): ductus closure: 3 doses separated by 12-24 hrs; 1st dose: 0.2 mg/kg; 2nd and 3rd doses depend on age: < 48 hrs: 0.1 mg/kg 2-7 days: 0.2 mg/kg > 7 days: 0.25 mg/kg	• GI ulceration or bleeding • renal dysfunction • inhibits platelet aggregation • cross-reaction between aspirin and indomethacin	• inhibits cyclooxygenase • anti-inflammatory, analgesic and antipyretic • anti-pyretic effect in Hodgkin's disease
Insulin: diabetic ketoacidosis: bolus: regular insulin 0.1 unit/kg IV infusion: regular insulin 0.1 unit/kg/hr IV hyperkalemia: regular insulin 0.15 unit/kg IV with 0.5 gm/kg glucose	• allergic reaction: rash • hypoglycemia • insulin binds to plastic IV administration materials	• stimulates transport of metabolites (esp. glucose) and ions (esp. K^+ and Mg^{++} through membranes • stimulates glycogen and fat synthesis • inhibits glycogenolysis and lipolysis • regular IV onset: ½-1 hr semilente SC onset: ½-1hr NPH SC onset: 1-2hrs
Isoproterenol (Isuprel): For hypotension, bradycardia, refractory bronchospasm: infusion: 0.05 µg/kg/min IV increase q4min by 0.05 µg/kg/min and titrate to effect Preparation: see dobutamine	• tachycardia, tachyarrhythmias	• β_1 and β_2 adrenergic agonists

Ketamine:
intubation: 1-2 mg/kg IV, 6-10 mg/kg IM;
sedation: 1/6 of the above doses

- releases endogenous catecholamines: ↑ BP and HR
- direct myocardial depressant
- hallucinations (give benzodiazepines concomitantly)
- ↑ intraocular and intracranial pressure
- lowers seizure threshold
- stimulates salivary secretions (give atropine concomitantly)

- site of action? cortex and limbic systems
- provides cardiovascular stability

Labetolol (Trandate):
For Hypertension:
adults: 5-10 mg IV bolus titrated to effect acutely
children: 0.07-0.15 mg/kg IV

- α to β receptor blockade (ratio 1:3 to 1:7)
- rashes
- see propranolol

- selective α_1-antagonism
- nonselective β-antagonism
- inhibits re-uptake of norepinephrine into nerve terminals

Newborns	6 mos	2 yrs	3 yrs	10 yrs	Adults
3 kg	7 kg	12 kg	14 kg	32 kg	70 kg

Lidocaine: For Ventricular arrhythmias, Intubation: 1-1.5 mg/kg IV or intratracheal; IV infusion: 20-50 μg/kg/min Preparation: see dobutamine	• can suppress a diseased SA node • agitation (serum level: 5 μg/ml) • hearing disturbances • convulsions (serum level > 7 μg/ml)	• blocks some of the stimulation of laryngoscopy and tracheal intubation • decreases slope of phase 4 depolarization of Purkinje fibers • increases ventricular fibrillation threshold • treats ventricular arrhythmias
Lorazepam (Ativan): status epilepticus, sedation: 0.03-0.05 mg/kg/dose PO, IV, IM	• see Diazepam	• see Diazepam
Mannitol: cerebral edema: 0.25 gm/kg/dose IV	• fluid overload by expansion of the extracellular space esp. in heart failure and anuria • can accumulate and raise the serum osmolarity to dangerous levels > 340 mosm/kg	• osmotically active agent • ? free radical scavenger
Meperidine (Demerol): 1-1.5 mg/kg/dose PO, IM, IV, SC q3h; max 100 mg q3h	• see morphine • convulsions, blocked by naloxone are mediated by normeperidine • neonates do not clear the drug well • respiratory depression	• see morphine • interacts with the κ-receptors more than morphine • may increase heart rate

Methadone (Dolphine): 0.1 mg/kg/dose q8-12h PO, IV*, IM, SC. *Although not approved for IV use, it is routinely done.	•antitussive •constipation •sedation •miosis •biliary spasm •respiratory depression
Metaproterenol (Metaprel, Alupent) Status asthmaticus: Nebulized: 0.2-0.3 ml of 5% sol in 2.5 ml NS q 30 min Aerosol: 1-3 puffs q3h (650 µg/puff) Oral: 1.3-2.6 mg/kg/day q6-8h	•see isoproterenol •selective β_2-agonist •see isoproterenol
Methylprednisolone (Medrol, Solumedrol): anti-inflammatory: 0.4-1.6 mg/kg/day ÷ q6-12h IV asthma: load: 1-2 mg/kg/dose; maint: 0.5-4 mg/kg/dose q4-6h; IV max 250 mg/dose q4h spinal cord trauma: 30 mg/kg/dose IV bolus followed by 5.4 mg/kg/hr IV	•see hydrocortisone •see hydrocortisone •5 times the antiinflammatory and half the sodium retaining potency of hydrocortisone
Midazolam (Versed): Sedation: parenteral: 0.05-0.3 mg/kg q1-2h IM, IV oral: 1 mg/kg PO	•see diazepam •see diazepam •water soluble

Newborns	6 mos	2 yrs	3 yrs	10 yrs	Adults
3 kg	7 kg	12 kg	14 kg	32 kg	70 kg

Morphine Sulfate: 0.1-0.2 mg/kg/dose SC, IV or IM q3-4h	• sedation, nausea, vomiting, respiratory depression, miosis, constipation, biliary spasm, muscular rigidity in high doses • suppresses the cough reflex • vasodilation • histamine release causing hypotension and bronchospasm • withdrawal symptoms after prolonged use	• μ- and κ- agonist, little effect on σ-receptors • μ-effects: supraspinal analgesia, respiratory depression, euphoria, physical dependence • κ-effect: spinal analgesia, sedation, miosis • σ-effect: dysphoric hallucinations
Nafcillin (Staphcillin): newborns < 7 days: 40 mg/kg/day ÷ q12h IV, IM; > 7 days: 60 mg/kg/day ÷ q6-8h; children: 100-200 mg/kg/day ÷ q4h IV; adults: 4-12 gm/day ÷ q4h IV	• see penicillin	• see penicillin • resistant to penicillinase • active against staphylococcal infections • good bile and CSF concen.
Naloxone (Narcan): 5-10 μg/kg/dose IM or IV q 3-5 min	• can precipitate a withdrawal syndrome • can cause loss of analgesia • duration of narcotic may exceed duration of naloxone	• μ-receptor antagonist • some antagonism to κ- and σ-receptors
Neostigmine: Reversal of neuromuscular blockade: 0.06-0.07 mg/kg IV; max 3 mg Anticholinergic (e.g., atropine) should be given concomitantly	• salivation, lacrimation, diarrhea, vomiting, bradycardia, bronchiolar and ureteral contraction	• inhibits acetylcholinesterase

Nifedipine: Hypertension: 0.25-0.5 mg/kg/dose q6-8h PO or sublingual; max 30 mg/dose (or 180 mg/day)	• hypotension, tachycardia, headaches, dizziness, palpitations	• calcium entry blocker • more potent vasodilator than verapamil • arterial dilation causes reflex changes of increased HR and cardiac output
Nitroglycerine: infusion: 1 µg/kg/min titrate up to effect <u>Preparation</u>: see Dobutamine	• venodilation • headaches, postural hypotension • absorbed onto the plastic of many IV administration sets	• increase c-GMP in smooth muscle • improves both myocardial oxygen supply and demand • less effective hypotensive agent than nitroprusside
Nitroprusside (Nipride, Nitropres): infusion: 0.5-8 µg/kg/min <u>Preparation</u>: see Dobutamine	• hypotension, sweating, headache • reflex tachycardia • methemoglobinemia • acute withdrawal can cause hypertensive crisis • cyanide toxicity with metabolic acidosis	• decreases both preload and afterload • direct vascular smooth muscle dilator

Newborns	6 mos	2 yrs	3 yrs	10 yrs	Adults
3 kg	7 kg	12 kg	14 kg	32 kg	70 kg

Norepinephrine (Levarterenol):
Hypotension:
  test dose: 0.1–0.2 μg/kg
  infusion: 0.05 μg/kg/min titrate up to effect
Preparation: see dobutamine
	•hypertension
	•cardiac arrhythmias
	•reflex bradycardia
		•β_1-agonist
		•little β_2 agonism
		•α-agonist

Pancuronium: For neuromuscular blockade: Intubation: 0.1–0.15 mg/kg IV	•tachycardia	Neuromuscular blockade prolonged by: •respiratory acidosis •myasthenic syndrome •metabolic alkalosis •local anesthetics •many antibiotics •magnesium •nitroglycerine •hypothermia

Penicillin G (potassium or sodium): ≤ 7 days: 50,000-150,000 U/kg/day ÷ q12h > 7 days: 75,000-200,000 U/kg/day ÷ q6-8h Children: 100,000-300,000 U/kg/day ÷ q6h IV, IM	• resistance • from most to least likely: rash, fever, bronchospasm, vasculitis, serum sickness, exfoliative dermatitis, Stevens-Johnson syndrome, anaphylaxis • less common: eosinophilia, interstitial nephritis	• interferes with cell wall synthesis • 1 mg = 1600 Units • 1.68 mEq Na^+ or K^+ per 1,000,000 units • activity against gram positive cocci, anaerobes, some Gram negatives • 5% of plasma concentration found in CSF in meningitis • Probenecid blocks tubular secretion
Pentobarbital (Nembutal): sedation: 2-6 mg/kg/dose PO, IV, IM coma induction: 10 mg/kg/dose x 1, then 1-4 mg/kg/hr	• apnea • hypotension • decreases cardiac output, cerebral blood flow, intracranial pressure • contraindicated in porphyrias • intra-arterial injection can cause loss of limb	• antianalgesic in subanesthetic doses • site of action: reticular activating system • inhibits synapses which are GABAergic

Newborns	6 mos	2 yrs	3 yrs	10 yrs	Adults
3 kg	7 kg	12 kg	14 kg	32 kg	70 kg

Phenobarbital (Luminal): sedation: 2-3 mg/kg/dose PO, IM, IV q8h seizure control: 15-25 mg/kg/dose IV; max 600 mg/day; chronic anticonvulsant: 4-6 mg/kg/day PO ÷ q12h	• see pentobarbital	• see pentobarbital
Phenylephrine (Neosynephrine): hypotension: 1-10 µg/kg IV repeat and titrate prn; then start with 0.05 µg/kg/min IV infusion and titrate SVT: 5-10 µg/kg/dose IV	• increased systemic vascular resistance • bradycardia (reflex)	• α₁ stimulation • may release norepinephrine
Phenytoin (Dilantin): seizures: 15-20 mg/kg IV; anti-arrhythmic: 2-4 mg/kg IV; max 500 gm maximum administration rate: 1 mg/kg/min	• cardiac arrhythmias, hypotension • megaloblastic anemia, neutropenia, leukopenia, lymphadenopathy • gingival hyperplasia, dermatitis • nystagmus, ataxia, diplopia, vertigo • inhibition of ADH release	• for treatment of all seizures except absence seizures • stabilizes neural membranes • below toxic levels - no CNS effects • follow QT on ECG while loading
Physostigmine (Antilirium): Antihistamine or anticholinergic overdose: children < 5 yrs: 0.5 mg IV q5min; max 2.0 mg; ≥ 5 yrs: 1-2 mg IV; max 4 mg/30 min	• salivation • lacrimation • seizures Atropine will reverse these toxic side effects	• inhibits cholinesterase • crosses the blood brain barrier See Chapter 11
Pipercillin (Pipracil): 75-300 mg/kg/day ÷ q4-6h IV, IM; max 24 gm/day	• see penicillin	• see penicillin • activity against Klebsiella and Pseudomonas

| | Prednisolone: anti-inflammatory & asthma: 0.5-2 mg/kg/day IV, IM ÷ q6h physiologic replacement: 4-5 mg/day ÷ q12h | •see hydrocortisone •4 times the anti-inflammatory effects and 0.8 times the sodium retaining effects as hydrocortisone | •supersensitivity to catecholamines •change in mental status •contraindicated in depressed patients, peptic ulcer disease |
| | Procainamide (Pronestyl): IM: 20-30 mg/kg/day ÷ q4-6h; adults: 1 gm/dose x 1, then 250 mg q3h; max 4 gm/day IV load: 2 mg/kg/dose IV over 5 min; adults: 100 mg IV over 2-4 min q5 min titrated to control of dysrhythmia maintenance: 20-80 µg/kg/min; adults: max 8 gm/day | •used for PVCs, also moderate activity on atrial flutter/fibrillation •decreases automaticity, V_max, action potential amplitude •prolongs action potential and effective refractory period •prolongs QRS, QT •usually digitalization •should commence prior to quinidine initiation | •hypotension esp. when dose is > 600 mg •toxic level > 14 µg/ml •fewer vagolytic side effects than quinidine •discontinuation - same criteria as in quinidine •GI, CNS disturbances, agranulocytosis, SLE syndrome |

Newborns	6 mos	2 yrs	3 yrs	10 yrs	Adults
3 kg	7 kg	12 kg	14 kg	32 kg	70 kg

Propranolol (Inderal):
Supraventricular tachycardia: 0.01 mg/kg/dose IV, titrated up to 5 mg to effect
tetralogy spells: 0.15-0.25mg/kg/dose IV q15min, then 1-2 mg/kg/dose q6h PO; max single dose: 10 mg IV
thyrotoxicosis:
  for neonates: 2 mg/kg/day PO ÷ q6h;
  for adults: 1-3 mg/dose IV over 10 min, then 10-40 mg PO q6h
hypertension: 0.5 mg/kg/day ÷ q6-12h IV, PO
	•bronchospasm
	•augments the hypoglycemic actions of insulin by reducing the compensatory effect of sympathetic adrenal activation
	•bradycardia; propranolol contraindicated with concomitant verapamil use
	•nausea, vomiting
		•nonspecific β-antagonist
		•blocks renin release from juxtaglomerular sites
		•decreases spontaneous firing in atria and ectopic sites

Prostaglandin E₁ (PGE₁, alprostadil Prostin VR): initial: 0.05 μg/kg/min IV, titrated up to 0.2 μg/kg/min	•apnea, seizures, fever, flushing, bradycardia, hypotension, diarrhea •decreases platelet aggregation	•stimulates smooth muscle in low doses, but relaxes at higher doses •activates adenylate cyclase •pulmonary and ductal tissue relaxation
Protamine Sulfate: Heparin antidote: must be titrated to effect (e.g., against activated clotting time); max dose: 50 mg Start with 1 mg per 100 units heparin IV over 5 min	•dyspnea, flushing, bradycardia, hypotension avoided by slow central venous administration •? histamine release •hypersensitivity, esp. in fish allergic individuals	•combines with heparin ionically •1 mg protamine antagonizes 100 units of heparin

Quinidine: For practical purposes quinidine is only given PO, although it can be administered IM or IV under exceptional circumstances Test dose: 2 mg/kg <u>children</u>: 15-60 mg/kg/day ÷ q6h <u>adults</u>: 200-400 mg/dose q6-8h; 200-300 mg/dose q6-8h titrated to effect (ECG changes)	•level 14 μg/ml, 50% of patients will demonstrate toxic effects •syncope, sudden death •digitalization may be indicated prior to quinidine to ↑ AV block and prevent ↑ ventricular rate •hypotension, tachycardia, tinnitus, hearing loss, GI disturbances, fever, anaphylaxis, thrombocytopenia	•decreases action potential V_{max}, automaticity •prolongs action potential and refractory period •prolongs QRS •activity for atrial fibrillation and flutter, premature atrial contraction, premature ventricular contraction and reentry tachycardia •vagolytic and α-blocking properties
Ranitidine: <u>children</u>: 2-4 mg/kg/day ÷ q12h PO; 1-2 mg/kg/day ÷ q6-8h IV <u>adults</u>: 150 mg PO BID; 50 mg IV, IM q6-8h	•rare and minor side effects •small hepatic blood flow reductions causing accumulation of drugs which are metabolized in the liver	•H_2 histamine receptor blocker inhibits gastric secretion reducing gastric volume and increasing gastric pH
Ribavirin (Varazole) Administered by aerosol (20 mg/ml sterile water) for 12-18 hrs/day x 3-7 days	•can interfere with respirator function	•anti-viral agent for RSV

Newborns	6 mos	2 yrs	3 yrs	10 yrs	Adults
3 kg	7 kg	12 kg	14 kg	32 kg	70 kg

Rifampin:
prophylaxis for H flu:
  < 1 mo: 10 mg/kg/day qD x 4 days
  > 1 mo: 20 mg/kg/day qD x 4 days;
  max dose: 600 mg/day
prophylaxis for N. meningitis: 10 mg/kg/dose BID x 2 days
	• stains secretions (tears, urine) orange
	• may counteract the effects of oral birth control pills

Succinylcholine: Neuromuscular blockade, intubation: 1-1.5 mg/kg IV; 4 mg/kg IM	• atypical or absent pseudocholinesterase prolongs paralysis • hyperkalemia associated with burns, trauma and nerve damage > 24 hrs after injury • increases intraocular and intracranial pressures • malignant hyperthermia triggering agent
Sucralfate (Carafate): GI stress ulcer prophylaxis: adults 1 gm PO QID	• do not give antacids concomitantly, because sulfated sucrose and aluminum compounds polymerize at pH ≥ 4 • rare side effects • constipation • dry mouth • in uremic patients, increases serum aluminum and decreases serum phosphate levels
Terbutaline (Brethine, Bricanyl): SC: 0.005-0.01 mg/kg/dose; max 0.25 mg q15-20 min x 2 Inhalation: 2 inhalations q4h Nebulized: 0.2 mg/kg of a 1 mg/ml concentration diluted in 2.5 ml NS q20 min; max 10 mg	• see metaproterenol

Thiopental: deep sedation, general anesthesia, reduction of intracranial pressure: 1-7 mg/kg IV	• hypotension: direct myocardial depression; ganglionic blockade • not to be used in porphyrias • histamine release: hypotension, bronchospasm • intra-arterial injection can cause loss of limb • see pentobarbital	• potentiates both GABA and non-GABA induced chloride conductance • decreases cerebral metabolic rate and cerebral blood flow and volume, thus decreasing intracranial hypertension • see pentobarbital

Ticarcillin:
neonates:
  < 2 kg: 0-7 days: 150 mg/kg/day ÷ q12h IV;
  > 7 days: 225 mg/kg/day ÷ q8h IV;
  > 2 kg: 200-300 mg/kg/day ÷ q8h;
children: 200-300 mg/kg/day ÷ q4-6h IV, IM; max 30 gm/day
	• see penicillin	• see penicillin
		• each gram contains 5 mEq sodium
		• enhanced activity against pseudomonas

Tobramycin (Nebcin): 2.5 mg/kg/dose q8h IV Frequency for neonates: < 7 days (< 28 wks): q24h, 28-34 wks: q18h, term q12h); > 7 days (< 28 wks): q18h, 28-34 wks: q12h, term q8h)	• see gentamicin	• see gentamicin • enhanced activity against enterococci

Newborns	6 mos	2 yrs	3 yrs	10 yrs	Adults
3 kg	7 kg	12 kg	14 kg	32 kg	70 kg

Trimethoprim-sulfamethoxazole (TMP-SMX, Bactrim, Septra): severe infections and *Pneumocystis carinii* pneumonia; TMP dose: 20 mg/kg/day ÷ q6-8h PO, IV Pneumocystis prophylaxis: 10 mg/kg/day ÷ q12h PO, IV	•resistance •blood dyscrasias (especially megaloblastic anemia) •rashes very common •renal toxicity	•inhibits folic acid metabolism in bacteria (especially dihydrofolate reductase) •has good CNS penetration
Vancomycin (Vancocin): neonates of ≤ 7 days: 10 mg/kg/dose (< 1 kg: q24h; 1-2 kg: q18h; > 2 kg: q12h) ≥ 7 days: 10 mg/kg/dose (< 1 kg: q18h; 1-2 kg: q12h; > 2 kg: q8h) children: 10-15 mg/kg/dose q8h IV	•ototoxicity (especially at levels of 34 μg/ml) •nephrotoxicity •phlebitis •erythema "red neck syndrome"	•Gram positive activity •cell wall synthesis inhibition
Vasopressin (Pitressin) Diabetes Insipidus: IV dose; start at 0.0005 units/kg/hr, double the dose every 15 min to a maximal 0.02 units/kg/hr	•anaphylaxis, bronchospasm, urticaria •vertigo, "pounding" headache •water intoxication	•antidiuretic, ↑ reabsorption of water by the renal tubules
Vecuronium: Neuromuscular blockade, intubation: 0.1 mg/kg IV Rapid sequence intubation: 0.3 mg/kg	•non-depolarizing neuromuscular blocker •few cardiovascular effects, except possibly bradycardia when administered with fentanyl	•no histamine release •no ganglionic blockade •no effect on muscarinic cardiac receptors
Verapamil (Isoptine, Calan): supraventricular tachycardia: 1-15 yrs: 0.1-0.3 mg/kg IV; max 5 mg; adult 5-10 mg	•cardiovascular collapse when given in conjunction with a ß-blocker •hypotension •bradydysrhythmias •contraindicated in infants	•negative chronotropy and inotropy •calcium channel blocker •vascular smooth muscle relaxation

INDEX